BLUEPRINTS
Plastic Surgery

Blueprints **for your pocket!**

In an effort to answer a need for high yield review books for the elective rotations, Blackwell Publishing now brings you Blueprints in pocket size.

These new Blueprints provide the essential content needed during the elective rotations. They will also provide the basic content needed for USMLE Steps 2 and 3, or if you were unable to fit in the rotation, these new pocket-sized Blueprints are just what you need.

Each book will focus on the high yield essential content for the most commonly encountered problems of the specialty. Each book features these special appendices:

- Career and residency opportunities
- Commonly prescribed medications
- Self-test Q&A section

Ask for these at your medical bookstore or check them out online at www.blackwellmedstudent.com

Blueprints Dermatology
Blueprints Urology
Blueprints Pediatric Infectious Diseases
Blueprints Ophthalmology
Blueprints Plastic Surgery
Blueprints Orthopedics
Blueprints Hematology and Oncology
Blueprints Anesthesiology
Blueprints Infectious Diseases

BLUEPRINTS
Plastic Surgery

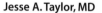

Jesse A. Taylor, MD
Fellow, Division of Reconstructive and Plastic Surgery
The Johns Hopkins Hospital and the University of Maryland
Baltimore, Maryland

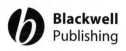

Blackwell
Publishing

© 2005 by Blackwell Publishing

Blackwell Publishing, Inc., 350 Main Street, Malden, Massachusetts
02148-5018, USA
Blackwell Publishing Ltd, 9600 Garsington Road, Oxford OX4 2DQ, UK
Blackwell Publishing Asia Pty Ltd, 550 Swanston Street, Carlton, Victoria
3053, Australia

04 05 06 07 5 4 3 2 1

ISBN: 1-4051-0446-5

Library of Congress Cataloging-in-Publication Data

Taylor, Jesse A.
    Blueprints plastic surgery/Jesse A. Taylor.
        p. ; cm.—(Blueprints)
    ISBN 1-4051-0446-5 (pbk. : alk. paper)   1. Surgery, Plastic—Handbooks,
manuals, etc.
    [DNLM: 1. Reconstructive Surgical Procedures—Outlines.
WO 18.2 T243b 2005]   I. Title: Plastic surgery.   II. Title.   III. Series.
RD118.T39 2005
617.9'5—dc22   2004019488

A catalogue record for this title is available from the British Library

Acquisitions: Beverly Copland
Development: Selene Steneck
Production: Debra Murphy
Illustrations: Electronic Illustrators Group
Cover design: Hannus Design Associates
Interior design: Mary McKeon
Typesetter: International Typesetting and Composition in Ft. Lauderdale, FL
Printed and bound by Capital City Press in Berlin, VT

For further information on Blackwell Publishing, visit our website:
www.blackwellmedstudent.com

Notice: The indications and dosages of all drugs in this book have been recommended in the medical literature and conform to the practices of the general community. The medications described do not necessarily have specific
approval by the Food and Drug Administration for use in the diseases and
dosages for which they are recommended. The package insert for each drug
should be consulted for use and dosage as approved by the FDA. Because
standards for usage change, it is advisable to keep abreast of revised recommendations, particularly those concerning new drugs.

To George and Marilyn Taylor

Contents

Contributors

Nia D. Banks, MD, PhD
Resident, Plastic and Reconstructive Surgery
Johns Hopkins Hospital
Baltimore, Maryland

Rachel Bluebond-Langner, MD
Resident, Plastic and Reconstructive Surgery
Johns Hopkins Hospital
Baltimore, Maryland

Thomas X. Hahm, MD
Fellow in Craniofacial Surgery
Division of Plastic and Reconstructive Surgery
Johns Hopkins Hospital
Baltimore, Maryland

Ryan Katz, MD
Resident, Plastic and Reconstructive Surgery
Johns Hopkins Hospital
Baltimore, Maryland

Marwan Khalifeh, MD
Resident, Plastic and Reconstructive Surgery
Johns Hopkins Hospital
Baltimore, Maryland

Michele Ann Manahan, MD
Resident, Plastic and Reconstructive Surgery
Johns Hopkins Hospital
Baltimore, Maryland

Gedge D. Rosson, MD
Resident, Plastic and Reconstructive Surgery
Johns Hopkins Hospital
Baltimore, Maryland

Subhro K. Sen, MD
Resident, Department of Surgery
Indiana University School of Medicine
Indianapolis, Indiana

Reviewers

Alexander L. Ayzengart, MD
Resident in General Surgery
University of California San Francisco
San Francisco, California

Liza Cadnapaphornchai, MD
Emergency Medicine Intern
Denver Health Medical Center
Denver, Colorado

Mabelle Cohen, MD
Resident, Department of Surgery
University of South Alabama Medical Center
Mobile, Alabama

Sohail R. Shah, MD
Resident, Department of General Surgery
University of Missouri at Kansas City
Kansas City, Missouri

Clarence Williams, II
Class of 2004
University of Texas Medical Branch—Galveston
Galveston, Texas

Preface

Blueprints have become the standard for medical students to use during their clerkship rotations and sub-internships and as a review book for taking the USMLE Steps 2 and 3.

Blueprints initially were only available for the five main specialties: medicine, pediatrics, obstetrics and gynecology, surgery, and psychiatry. Students found these books so valuable that they asked for Blueprints in other topics and so family medicine, emergency medicine, neurology, cardiology, and radiology were added.

In an effort to answer a need for high yield review books for the elective rotations, Blackwell Publishing now brings you Blueprints in pocket size. These books are developed to provide students in the shorter, elective rotations, often taken in 4th year, with the same high yield, essential contents of the larger Blueprint books. These new pocket-sized Blueprints will be invaluable for those students who need to know the essentials of a clinical area but were unable to take the rotation. Students in physician assistant, nurse practitioner, and osteopath programs will find these books meet their needs for the clinical specialties.

Feedback from student reviewers gave high praise for this addition to the Blueprints brand. Each of these new books was developed to be read in a short time period and to address the basics needed during a particular clinical rotation. Please see the Series Page for a list of the books that will soon be in your bookstore.

Acknowledgments

I would like to thank my mentors in plastic surgery both at the Johns Hopkins Hospital and at the University of Maryland. All have contributed to my education more than they will ever know.

Specifically, I would like to thank Dr. Paul Manson, Dr. Nelson Goldberg, Dr. Adrian Barbul, Dr. Bob Spence, Dr. Maurice Nahabedian, Dr. Navin Singh, and Dr. Eduardo Rodriguez for their generous contributions to this book. They have added wisdom where there would otherwise have been little.

I would like to thank my family—Fannie Chance, George, Marilyn, Matt, Luke, Myra, and Phoenix—for all their support through the years. Lastly, I would like to thank Lisa Earnest, who has spent countless hours editing chapters and shepherding me through this project.

—Jesse A. Taylor, MD

Abbreviations

ABA	American Burn Association
ABG	arterial blood gas
AIDS	acquired immunodeficiency syndrome
ALT	anterolateral thigh (flap)
APL	abductor pollicis longus
ATLS	advanced trauma life support
BCC	basal cell carcinoma
BCT	breast conservation therapy
BEE	basal energy expenditure
b.i.d.	twice a day
BP	blood pressure
cc	cubic centimeter
CEA	cultured epithelial autografts
CFA	common femoral artery
CHF	congestive heart failure
CHgb	carboxyhemoglobin
cm	centimeters
CNS	central nervous system
COPD	chronic obstructive pulmonary disease
COX-2	cyclooxygenase-2
CT	computerized tomography
CTS	carpal tunnel syndrome
DCIS	ductal carcinoma *in situ*
DIEA	deep inferior epigastric artery
DIEP	deep inferior epigastric artery perforator
DIEP	deep inferior epigastric perforator (flap)
DIP	distal interphalangeal
DVT	deep vein thrombosis
ECRB	extensor carpi radialis brevis
ECRL	extensor carpi radialis longus
ECU	extensor carpi ulnaris
EDM	extensor digiti minimi
EGF	epidermal growth factor
EIP	extensor indicis proprius
EMG	electromyography
EPB	extensor pollicis brevis
EPL	extensor pollicis longus
ET	endotracheally
FCR	flexor carpi radialis

FCU	flexor carpi ulnaris
FDA	U.S. Food and Drug Administration
FDP	flexor digitorum profundus
FDS	flexor digitorum superficialis
FGF	fibroblast growth factor
FPL	flexor pollicis longus
FTSG	full thickness skin grafts
GI	gastrointestinal
hGH	human growth hormone
hr	hour
ICU	intensive care unit
IGF-1	insulin-like growth factor 1
IL-1	interleukins
IM	intramuscularly
IMA	internal mammary artery
IV	intravenous
kg	kilogram
LCIS	lobular carcinoma *in situ*
LDH	lactate dehydrogenase
LDM	latissimus dorsi muscle
LGV	lymphogranuloma venereum
M	distant metastasis
MCP	metacarpophalangeal
MMF	maxillomandibular fixation
MRI	magnetic resonance imaging
MRM	modified radical mastectomy
MRSA	methicillin resistant *staphylococcus aureus*
N	nodal involvement
NAC	nipple areolar complex
NCV	nerve conduction velocity
NRMP	National Residency Matching Program
NSAID	nonsteroidal anti-inflammatory drug
PABA	para-aminobenzoic acid
PCA	patient controlled analgesia
PCN	penicillin
PDGF	platelet derived growth factor
PIN	posterior interosseous nerve
PIP	proximal interphalangeal
PMN	polymorphonuclear leukocyte
q.d.	once a day
SC	subcutaneously
SCC	squamous cell carcinoma
SFA	superficial femoral artery
SGAP	superior gluteal artery perforator (flap)
SIRS	systemic inflammatory response syndrome
SJS	Stevens-Johnson syndrome
SMAS	superficial musculoaponeurotic system
STSG	split thickness skin grafts

T	tumor size
TBSA	total body surface area
TENS	toxic epidermal necrolysis
TGF-α	transforming growth factor-alpha
TGF-β	transforming growth factor-beta
Tis	tumor *in situ*
TNF	tumor necrosis factor
TNM	tumor, node, metastasis
TRAM	transverse rectus abdominis myocutaneous (flap)
TRAMP	transverse rectus abdominis musculocutaneous perforator (flap)
UAL	ultrasound assisted liposuction
UV	ultraviolet

Basic Techniques

Rachel Bluebond-Langner, MD

Suture

The purpose of suture is to maintain apposition of tissues while they heal. The issues in choosing a suture are where in the body the suture is being used, how long the suture is intended to last, and the tensile strength of the suture, **that is**, the amount of force a knotted suture can withstand before breaking (Table 1-1).

■ Suture Permanence

Absorbable suture is made either of natural material that undergoes enzymatic digestion or synthetic material that is hydrolyzed by water. The rate of absorption varies with the type of material used. Fever and a moist environment will increase rate of absorption. Absorbable sutures are useful when suture removal may be difficult (**e.g.**, in a child or an unreliable patient). Absorbable suture is also used in environments with high crystalloid concentrations that may precipitate stones like the urinary or biliary tract.

Permanent suture is made from various plastics. It becomes encapsulated in fibrous scar tissue over time, making it inert. This is useful in slow healing tissues such as fascia and tendons. Patients with a history of scar hypertrophy or keloid formation benefit from the use of nonabsorbable suture that is removed early.

■ Monofilament versus Braided

Monofilament sutures are single strands that encounter less resistance as they pass through tissue and incite relatively little inflammation. However, they have less tensile strength than a braided suture of the same caliber, and break more easily if crushed or crimped.

Braided or polyfilament sutures are woven strands that provide greater tensile strength, flexibility, and pliability. Their downside is a greater inflammatory reaction and an increased potential for bacterial seeding, as the weave of a polyfilament suture can be thought of as a nest for bacteria.

TABLE 1-1 Common Suture Materials

	Material	Loss of Tensile strength	Inflammatory Reaction	Absorbed	Common Uses
Absorbable					
Gut					
Plain	Sheep intestine	7–10 days	Moderate	2 mo	Superficial vessels, closure of tissues that heal rapidly (buccal mucosa) and require minimal support
Chromic	Treated with chromium salt	10–14 days	Moderate, but less	3 mo	
Polylactic acid (Vicryl), polyglycolic acid (Dexon)	Synthetic polyfilament	4–5 wk	Minimal	3 mo	Dermis, fat, muscle
Polyglyconate (Maxon, Moncryl)	Synthetic monofilament	3–4 wk	Minimal	3–4 mo	Subcuticular closure and soft tissue approximation
Polydioxanone (PDS)	Synthetic monofilament	8 wk	Minimal	6 mo	Muscle, fascia
Nonabsorbable					
Polypropylene (Prolene)	Polymer of propylene	Years*	Minimal		Fascia, muscle, vessels
Nylon (Surgilon, Nurolon)	Polyamide	Years*	Minimal		Skin; drains; microsurgical anastomoses
Silk	Raw silk spun by silk worm	1 yr	Intense		Tie off vessels; bowel
Staples	Iron–chromium–nickel		Minimal		Skin

*With reoperation, Prolene and nylon remain present, but they decompose slightly.

■ Caliber

The caliber of suture is described with a measurement system that is stated in 0's (i.e., 5-0 is 00000). The number of 0's is determined by how many suture diameters are added to make 1 mm, so a 2-0 suture has twice the diameter of a 4-0 suture. Generally, surgeons use the smallest caliber suture capable of maintaining tissue apposition. Some suture is coated to decrease drag through tissue, and the coating, although it increases caliber, is not considered when naming its caliber.

■ Needles

Sutures come with or without a needle. Sutures without needles are called "ties." Needles have three components: the eye, the body, and the point. The eye of the needle is the way the needle is attached to the suture. The closed eye is similar to a household sewing needle. The **swagged** eye joins the suture and needle in continuity and is the most common and convenient since it is preloaded. **"Pop off"** sutures are a type of swagged suture in which the suture separates from the needle with a small but concerted effort. The body of the needle is the portion grasped by the needle driver. The configuration of the body ranges from straight to U-shaped. The point of the needle can be either **"cutting"** or **"tapered."** Cutting needles have two opposing cutting edges and are used to penetrate tough tissue such as skin or fibrous scar tissue. A tapered needle has a smooth barrel that tapers to a sharp point to allow smooth passage of the needle through tissue like fascia, vessels, and muscle.

Instruments

■ Needle Driver

The needle driver is used to pass a curved needle through tissue. The jaws that grip the needle have a variety of surfaces: smooth (which allow the needle to wobble in the holder) or granular (which grasp the needle more securely). The strength of the jaws of the needle driver should be proportional to the size of the needle. The length of the driver should be proportionate to the depth in which the surgeon is working, that is, shorter driver for skin, longer if working in a cavity.

■ Forceps

Forceps allow the nondominant hand to grasp and stabilize tissues. There are many types, and each has its specific use. **Adsons** come with or without "teeth" on the tip for picking up skin. **Adson-Browns** have a row of teeth on the tip for picking up deeper tissue such as the dermis, fascia, or fat. The **Debakey** forceps has a flat tip with fine ridges for picking up vessels and other deep tissue. Forceps are held like a pencil so that tissue can be manipulated gently.

■ Scalpels

Scalpels are sharp knives used to make surgical incisions. They come in a variety of shapes and sizes, the most common of which are the #10 blade and the #15 blade. The "belly" of the larger #10 blade is used to make long, sweeping incisions, whereas the tip of the smaller #15 blade is used to make fine, angled incisions.

Techniques

A fine-line scar is achieved by **minimizing tension**, **everting wound edges**, and **gently approximating tissues**. All sutures incite some degree of inflammatory response. Therefore, minimizing the amount of suture material reduces inflammation and consequently scarring. Early removal of superficial skin stitches can improve the scar as well. Cross-hatching in skin results from prolonged pressure, a combination of excessive tension and late suture removal. Table 1-2 contains suggestions for suture repair of selected soft tissue injuries.

■ Continuous

This fast suturing technique in which the needle repeatedly passes from superficial to deep on one side of the incision and deep to superficial on the other side uses a single suture. The tension is distributed along the full length of suture and is often used on the fascia and skin (Figure 1-1). **Continuous locking**, a variation on the theme, is done by passing the needle back through the loop with every stitch. It achieves better hemostasis and a more watertight seal, and is especially useful in the richly vascularized scalp.

■ Interrupted

There are various types of interrupted suture closure. In **simple interrupted** closure, the needle enters one side of the incision, passes through the wound, exits on the other side of the incision, and is tied down (Figure 1-2a). In the face, stitches are usually placed 5 to 7 mm apart and 1 to 2 mm from the edge. The **simple interrupted** stitch is ideal for apposition of tissues, but care must

TABLE 1-2 Suggested Suture Repair of Soft Tissue Injuries

Location	Suture Material	Closure Technique	Dressing	Comments
Face	5-0 or 6-0 nonabsorbable monofilament (in young children: 5-0 chromic)	Simple, interrupted; layered closure if full thickness	Bacitracin	Carefully examine for underlying injury (facial nerve, parotid duct); early suture removal recommended (3–5 days)
Scalp	Staples or 3-0 monofilament nonabsorbable	Running or running-locking	Bacitracin	Hemostasis is the key—avoid loose closure
Lip	4-0 gut for oral mucosa and wet vermilion; 6-0 monofilament nonabsorbable for dry vermilion	Simple interrupted; may use running; horizontal mattress helpful in oral mucosa	Bacitracin	Most important aesthetic concern is lining up the "red line" and "white line" of the lip
Eyebrow	5-0 synthetic absorbable	Inverted dermal followed by running subcuticular	Bacitracin	NEVER shave the eyebrow; excise parallel to direction of hair follicles (eyebrows may not grow back)
Eyelid	8-0 silk (skin) 8-0 Vicryl (tarsus)	Simple interrupted	None	Align lid margin and gray line perfectly
Hands	3-0 or 4-0 nonabsorbable monofilament	Simple, running, horizontal mattress; single layer closure is the rule	Dry dressing; frequently splinted	Must examine for concomitant injuries to bone, nerves, vessels, etc.

(Continued)

TABLE 1-2 Suggested Suture Repair of Soft Tissue Injuries (Contd.)

Location	Suture Material	Closure Technique	Dressing	Comments
Nailbed	5-0 chromic	Simple interrupted	Splint between cuticle and nail matrix to prevent adhesions	Original nail, if available, makes an ideal splint and dressing
Ear	5-0 synthetic absorbable for cartilage; 6-0 monofilament nonabsorbable for skin	Simple interrupted	Bolster dressing to prevent hematoma or seroma formation	Débride all cartilage that appears nonviable
Trunk	2-0 to 4-0 synthetic absorbable in dermis; skin staples or 3-0 synthetic absorbable	Inverted dermal; running subcuticular in skin	Dry dressing taken down 2 days postsurgery and wound left open to air	Internal organ damage must be ruled out

These suggestions for students are not controversial. Experienced surgeons may suggest alternatives that are equally acceptable.

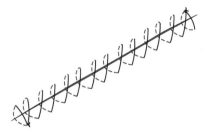

Figure 1-1 • Continuous "running" simple stitch.

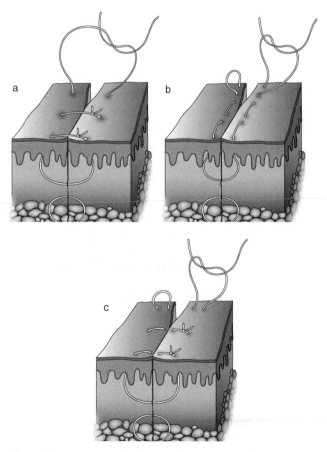

Figure 1-2 • (a) Simple interrupted stitch. (b) Horizontal mattress stitch. (c) Vertical mattress stitch.

be taken to enter and exit the skin perpendicularly and at the same level. Otherwise, it is difficult to evert wound edges. The **horizontal mattress stitch**, in which two simple, opposing passes of the needle are thrown and fastened, was developed to assist in eversion of wound edges (Figure 1-2b). The **vertical mattress stitch** (Figure 1-2c) both everts and apposes skin well.

Tradition suggests that interrupted sutures are better for wounds that are liable to dehisce, such as those at high risk for infection or those in patients on steroid therapy. That said, there are no data proving a benefit of interrupted closure over running closure. Surgeons have debated the point for years, and it is easy to find die-hards on both sides of the issue. Multiple studies comparing different suture closure techniques have demonstrated no difference in strength, infection rates, or aesthetics.

■ Subcuticular

A running **subcuticular stitch** in which the needle passes parallel to the incision at the dermal–epidermal junction, alternating sides (Figure 1-3), is another method of apposing the epidermis. Its advantages include speed of closure and suture invisibility. If absorbable suture material is used, no suture removal is necessary.

■ Buried Knots

In plastic surgery you will often see the dermal layer closed first with simple interrupted sutures, burying the knot. In order to bury the knot, the first pass of the needle must be from deep in

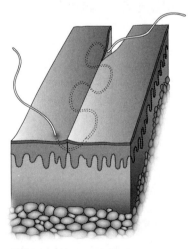

Figure 1-3 • Subcuticular closure.

the wound to the superficial surface and then superficial to deep on the opposite side. The interrupted dermal stitch with a buried knot reduces tension on the epidermis, reduces the amount of dead space, and helps to approximate the skin edges. Burying the knot helps to minimize the chance of developing a draining sinus tract along sutures.

Basic Laceration Management

■ Immunization

One should consider tetanus immunization following any trauma in which the skin barrier is broken. Immunity lasts approximately 10 years, so if a patient has received a shot within a 10-year period, additional prophylaxis is not warranted.

■ Débridement and Irrigation

Copious irrigation with sterile saline will help to remove foreign debris and clot from the wound bed. Sharp débridement is often needed to rid the wound of devitalized tissues.

■ Antiseptic Technique

Clean the skin around the wound with antiseptic—Betadine or chlorhexadine will suffice. These agents are damaging to exposed tissue and should be kept out of the wound. Cut hair as needed, but never shave eyebrows because they occasionally fail to grow back.

■ Wound Exploration

Before closure, a careful neurovascular examination and local wound exploration should be undertaken to diagnose and treat any injury to nerves, tendons, joints, or other structures in anatomic proximity. Often further diagnostic studies like x-rays and CT scans are necessary to pick up occult fractures.

■ Local Anesthesia

Anesthetize the wound prior to any manipulation. Lidocaine either with or without epinephrine (epinephrine is contraindicated in areas where ischemia may become an issue, i.e., digits, tip of penis, tip of nose) provides reliable, short-term local anesthesia.

■ Closure

The following are the fundamentals of surgical wound closure popularized by Dr. William Stewart Halsted in the early 20th century. They are still valid.

1. Careful hemostasis
2. Gentle handling of tissues
3. Tension-free closure
4. Placement of incisions along natural skin folds and relaxed skin tension lines
5. Eversion of wound edges

Dressing

A dressing should provide a clean, warm, moist environment for maximal wound healing. It should protect the wound during the period of reepithelialization, usually 48 hours. Surgeon preference dictates choice of dressing, and there are few data comparing surgical dressings. The following is a brief list of dressing materials commonly used by plastic surgeons:

1. Antibacterial ointments (e.g., Bacitracin, Neosporin) provide a warm, moist environment. Transparent, allowing for easy inspection of the wound. Usually applied twice daily
2. Vaseline impregnated gauze (e.g., Xeroform, Adaptic) moistens the incision. Usually applied beneath dry gauze and left in place for 48 hours.
3. Dry gauze (e.g., 4 × 4's, ABD pads) protects the wound and absorbs excess moisture. Cheap and effective.
4. Occlusive dressings (e.g., Tegaderm, OpSite) provide a warm, moist environment. Transparent, allowing for easy wound inspection.

Excising Skin Lesions

- **Wedge**: Any lesion close to an edge such as the lip, the nose, the eyelid or the ear can be excised with a wedge or a "V" and then closed primarily (Figure 1-4a).
- **Circular**: A circular pattern permits minimal tissue excision and is useful in areas such as the nose or ear where preservation of the skin is necessary. Circular excision usually requires skin graft or flap closure (Figure 1-4b).
- **Ellipse**: An elliptical pattern allows for simple excision and easy primary closure on nearly any surface of the body. The ideal geometry with regard to both tissue preservation and aesthetics is a length four times the width (Figure 1-4c).

Closing Simple Skin Defects

Some wounds are not amenable to primary closure, and there are a variety of ways to rearrange local tissue in order to close these

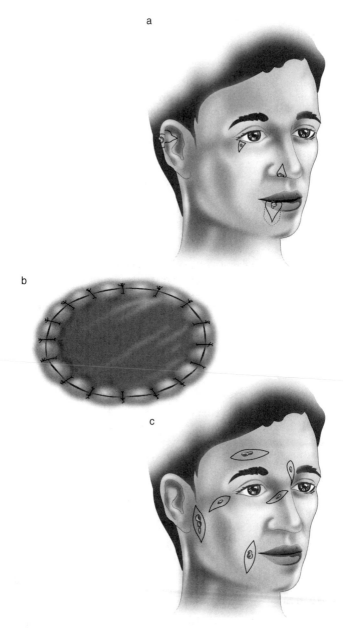

Figure 1-4 • (a) Wedge excision. (b) Circular excision with skin graft reconstruction. (c) Elliptical excision.

defects. The descriptions of these techniques may appear complicated, but the geometry is clear in the accompanying figures.

■ Pivoting Flaps

Pivoting flaps are skin and subcutaneous tissue that rotate through an arc about a fixed pivot point (Figure 1-5a). The effective length of the flap shortens as it rotates through the arc. The radius of the arc or edge of the flap is the point of maximal tension and can be back-cut to ease tension. All pivoting flaps require loose skin and are thus more successful in older patients.

- **Rotation flap**: This semicircular flap rotates across an arc into the defect. The length of base is generally four to five times the length of the defect (Figure 1-5b).
- **Transposition flap**: This rectangular flap rotates about a pivot point into an adjacent tissue defect. The greater the angle of rotation, the shorter it becomes (Figure 1-5c).
- **Interpolation flap**: This flap is rotated into nearby but not adjacent tissue. A skin bridge is created that must pass under or over the intervening fixed tissue.
- **Bilobed flap**: This flap has two lobes designed at right angles to one another. The primary flap rotates into the initial defect while the secondary flap closes the donor site. The secondary flap is designed to be half the diameter of the primary flap (Figure 1-5d).

■ Advancement Flaps

These flaps are also composed of skin, subcutaneous tissue, and a blood supply but are "advanced" directly into a defect without rotation or lateral movement. The degree of advancement is dependent on the skin's elasticity. Two common patterns are:

- **Single pedicle**: A square or rectangular pedicle is advanced forward into a defect.
- **V-Y advancement flap**: A triangular or "V" flap is advanced directly without rotation and closed to form the pattern of a "Y." This is useful in lengthening the nasal columella, correcting notches in the lip, or closing soft tissue defects such as the donor site of a skin flap (Figure 1-6).

■ Z-plasty

Z-plasty is a classic technique used by plastic surgeons to gain length. It can be used to correct scar contracture, especially when

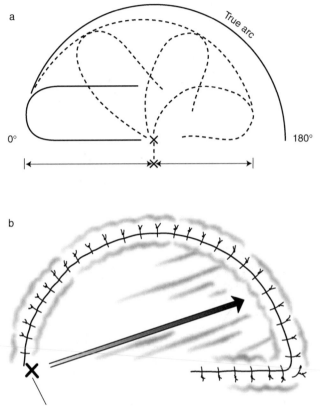

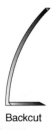

Backcut

Figure 1-5 • (a) Pivot flap. (b) Rotational flap. *(Continued)*

c

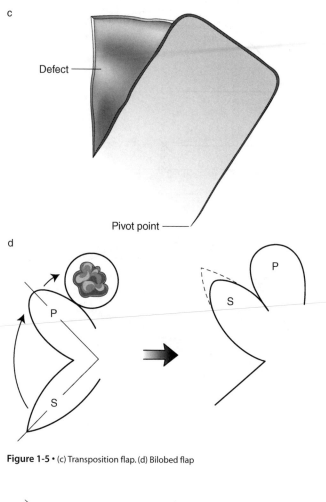

d

Figure 1-5 • (c) Transposition flap. (d) Bilobed flap

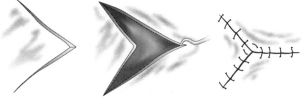

Figure 1-6 • V-Y advancement flap.

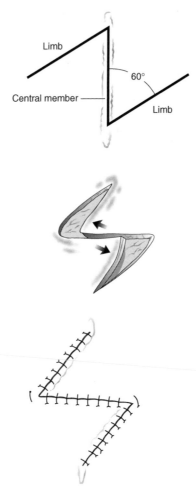

Figure 1-7 • Z-plasty.

it affects function. It allows for a gain in length and a change in direction so that mobility improves. Two triangles are juxtaposed to one another about a central axis (Figure 1-7). All limbs of the "Z" must be equal in length. The angle between limbs can vary from 30 to 90 degrees based on the desired gain in length. The standard Z-plasty uses 60 degree angles, which gives a 75% increase in length. The less acute the angle, the greater the gain in length but the more tension placed on the suture line. For example, 30 degree angles produce a 25% gain in length, whereas 90 degree angles produce a 120% gain in length. The pattern is oriented about a central line that lies in the direction of desired gain in length. Thus, length is gained along the central axis.

W-plasty

W-plasty is similar to Z-plasty. It, too, changes the direction of a scar, but unlike Z-plasty it does not lead to large gains in length. Serial triangles interdigitate about the original central scar.

2

Wound Healing

Jesse A. Taylor, MD

A wound is any disruption of normal anatomic relationships between tissues. The ability to heal wounds by forming scar is essential to our survival. Facilitating wound healing is the principal aim of plastic surgery, and derangement of healing is the leading cause of morbidity in plastic surgery patients.

When injured, the body begins to heal immediately and the wound continues to remodel throughout life. Medical science is just beginning to understand this process on a cellular and molecular level.

Molecular and Cellular Mediators of Healing

■ Collagen

Collagen is the most abundant family of proteins in the human body, providing strength and integrity for all tissues. Immediately following injury, exposed collagen comes into contact with blood and promotes platelet aggregation, activation, and release of chemotactic factors involved in the response to injury. Later, collagen becomes the foundation of the wound extracellular matrix, providing tensile strength to the wound. Of the many types of collagen, type I is the most common and is found throughout the body. Immature scar has an abundance of type III collagen which dissipates as the scar matures. Mature scar has a type I to type III collagen ratio of 4:1.

■ Platelets

Platelets are the first of the inflammatory mediators to reach a wound. They are essential for clot formation as well as chemotaxis. Their alpha granules contain growth factors like platelet-derived growth factor (PDGF), transforming growth factor-beta (TGF-β), and platelet factor IV, which attract and activate fibroblasts, endothelial cells, and macrophages. Platelets also contain dense bodies that store vasoactive amines, like histamine, which vasodilate and increase microvascular permeability.

■ Polymorphonuclear Leukocytes

PMNs are also early responders in the inflammatory cascade. Their primary responsibility is to remove bacteria and foreign debris from the wound, thereby helping to prevent infection. They add little else to the healing process. Studies suggest that wound healing proceeds normally in the absence of PMNs.

■ Macrophages

Macrophages are key players in wound healing. They achieve high concentrations in the wound by 48 hours postinjury and remain throughout the inflammatory phase of wound healing, actively participating in débridement. They promote angiogenesis and release chemokines that attract fibroblasts to the wound, thus regulating the synthesis and deposition of collagen.

■ Growth Factors

Growth factors are polypeptides or glycoproteins that are synthesized by one cell for communication with another. In a healing wound they are responsible for the orderly procession of cells into a wound, the proliferation of cells, and the production of extracellular proteins (Table 2-1). In short, their careful orchestration is responsible for normal, efficient healing. Similarly, alterations in their production and responsiveness contribute to proliferative disorders, such as excessive scarring and neoplasm, as well as impaired wound healing.

■ Lymphocytes

T-lymphocytes reach the wound bed by day 3 postinjury, and play a minor role in fibroblast proliferation and angiogenesis. Their role in wound healing is poorly understood. Interestingly, AIDS patients do not exhibit delayed or deficient wound healing.

■ Fibroblasts

Fibroblasts begin to migrate into a wound bed by day 4 postinjury, and are the predominant cell type in the wound by day 7. Fibroblasts synthesize collagen and glycosaminoglycans, which increases in a linear fashion for 2 to 3 weeks. As a wound achieves collagen equilibrium, the number of fibroblasts begins to decrease.

■ Myofibroblasts

Myofibroblasts are specialized fibroblasts equipped with cytoplasmic microfilaments similar to smooth muscle cells. They act to close the gap created by a wound, a process known as wound

■ TABLE 2-1 Growth Factors in Wound Healing

Growth Factor	Source	Target and Functions
Epidermal growth factor (EGF)	Platelets, macrophages	Promotes epithelial cell and fibroblast proliferation
Fibroblast growth factors (FGFs)	Fibroblasts, endothelial cells, epithelial cells	Cellular proliferation; stimulate matrix deposition, wound contraction, and angiogenesis
Human growth hormone (hGH)	Pituitary	Anabolic steroid; hypothetical anti-aging effect promotes release of IGF-1—the active hormone
Insulin-like growth factor 1 (IGF-1)	Fibroblasts, liver	Stimulates synthesis of ground substance and collagen; fibroblast proliferation
Interleukins (IL-1, etc.)	Macrophages, lymphocytes, many other cells and tissues	Important role in chemotaxis; fibroblast proliferation
Platelet-derived growth factor (PDGF)	Platelets, macrophages, endothelial cells, fibroblasts, smooth muscle cells	Chemotaxis; fibroblast proliferation and collagen synthesis; angiogenesis
Transforming growth factor-α (TGF-α)	Activated macrophages, platelets, keratinocytes	Effects are similar to EGF; proliferation
Transforming growth factor-β (TGF-β)	All cells	Chemotaxis, fibroblast proliferation, actions of other growth factors
Tumor necrosis factor (TNF)	Macrophages, lymphocytes, mast cells	Fibroblast proliferation

contraction. They are present in a wound as long as there is a gap to be closed.

Time Sequence of Wound Healing

Wound healing proceeds as an orderly sequence of overlapping events. The process is identical regardless of the tissue involved. Generally, the process of scar formation that restores tensile strength is discussed in four phases: the coagulation phase, the inflammatory phase, the proliferative phase, and the maturation phase. Throughout the development of the scar, there is rejuvenation of the epithelial layer.

■ Coagulation

Tissue injury leads to extravasation of blood into the wound. Vasoconstriction occurs to limit blood loss. Platelets contact exposed collagens promoting aggregation and activation of chemotactic factors that attract PMNs, macrophages, and fibroblasts to the wound. The end product of both the intrinsic and extrinsic clotting cascade is fibrin, which provides a matrix into which inflammatory cells can migrate. In general, the coagulation phase of wound healing is brief, lasting only several minutes. The end product is blood clot on injured tissue.

■ Inflammation

The goal of the inflammatory phase of wound healing is to cleanse the wound and attract cells that will eventually rebuild injured tissue as scar. It is sometimes referred to as the "lag phase" of wound healing because wound strength does not return immediately during this phase. Following a brief period of vasoconstriction, histamine and other inflammatory mediators promote active vasodilation. There is a simultaneous increase in the permeability of vessel walls, allowing molecular and cellular mediators of inflammation to enter the wound. PMNs and macrophages begin débriding bacteria, debris, and necrotic tissue. In addition to aiding débridement, macrophages are the primary producers of growth factors responsible for both the production and proliferation of extracellular matrix by fibroblasts, proliferation of smooth muscle cells, and proliferation of endothelial cells resulting in angiogenesis. Generally, the inflammatory phase of wound healing begins within minutes of wounding and lasts about 1 week. Clinically, it is the phase of erythema and edema.

■ Proliferation

The proliferative, or fibroblastic, phase of wound healing begins about 2 to 3 days after wounding and proceeds for about 4 weeks. It consists of fibroblast proliferation, accumulation of ground substance, and collagen production. Within 24 hours of wounding, local mesenchymal cells are transformed into fibroblasts that migrate into the wound along a framework of fibrin fibers. They attach to the fibrin matrix of the clot, multiply, and begin producing glycosaminoglycans and fibrillar collagen. The glycosaminoglycans secreted are hydrated into an amorphous gel (ground substance) that plays an important role in the subsequent aggregation of collagen fibers. Collagen fibrils begin to appear as ground substance accumulates, and over a period of about 3 weeks collagen levels increase dramatically. As collagen levels rise, the number of fibroblasts in the wound decreases until the rates of collagen synthesis and degradation are the same—collagen homeostasis. Myofibroblasts produce contractile proteins that pull the edges of the wound together. Red, "beefy" granulation tissue is the result of the proliferative phase of wound healing.

■ Maturation

The maturation phase of wound healing begins approximately 3 weeks after wounding. It consists of collagen cross-linking, collagen remodeling, and wound contraction. By 3 weeks postinjury collagen homeostasis has been achieved, large numbers of new capillaries growing into the wound regress and disappear, and collagen fibers become organized in a pattern determined by local mechanical forces. The formerly indurated, raised, pruritic scar becomes a mature scar as the type III collagen is replaced by type I collagen until type I collagen is four times as prevalent. The ground substance, which plays such a key role in the proliferation phase, is degraded and dehydrated until the tissues resemble normal dermis. Myofibroblasts use specialized cytoplasmic microfilaments to close the wound gap in a process known as wound contraction. (Note: There is an important distinction between wound contraction and wound contracture. Wound contraction has been described above. Wound contracture is the pathologic process whereby an overabundance of collagen deposition leads to limitations of motion in a region.)

By 6 weeks postinjury, the wound reaches its maximal tensile strength, approximately 80% of its original strength. New collagen is deposited in more stable and permanent cross-links as the wound continues to remodel throughout life.

■ Epithelialization

Epithelialization refers to basal cell proliferation and epithelial migration occurring in a wound. The response of the epithelium to injury always follows the same sequence of mobilization, migration, mitosis, and cellular differentiation. In full-thickness wounds, epithelium at the wound margins begins to mobilize by detaching from the basement membrane and moving away from neighboring cells. Cells migrate across the wound as there is a loss of contact inhibition. As the leading edge cells migrate, the cells behind them mobilize and follow. Mitosis of basal epithelial cells occurs in order to provide cells for resurfacing. Once the wound gap is closed, epithelial cells resume the normal cellular differentiation from basal to surface layers. Clean surgical incisions usually achieve epithelialization within 48 hours.

In partial-thickness wounds, epithelialization proceeds from "epithelial islands" lining dermal structures rather than from the wound edges. Migration, mobilization, and mitosis proceed in similar fashion until the epithelial islands coalesce.

Factors Influencing Wound Healing

■ Oxygen

Oxygen is a critical nutrient in wound healing. Fibroblasts are oxygen sensitive, and both myofibroblast and collagen production can be stimulated by maintaining a wound in a state of hyperoxia. Oxygen supply controls the rate of epithelialization in normal and ischemic wounds. Collagen synthesis, matrix deposition, angiogenesis, and bacterial killing accelerate with elevation of arterial oxygen tension. Hyperbaric oxygen has been demonstrated to improve wound healing in chronically ischemic wounds. The most common cause of wound infection or failure of wounds to heal properly is deficient wound oxygenation.

■ Oxygen-Derived Free Radicals

Oxygen radicals cause cellular injury by degrading hyaluronic acid and collagen, destroying cell membranes, disrupting organelle membranes, and interfering with important protein enzyme systems. Oxygen free radicals form in the face of radiation, select chemical agents, ischemia, and inflammation.

■ Smoking

Nicotine acts via the sympathetic nervous system to produce vasoconstriction and limit blood flow necessary for distal perfusion. Smoke also contains high levels of carbon monoxide that tend to shift the oxygen-hemoglobin curve to the left and form carboxyhemoglobin. Both reduce oxygen supply to the wound.

■ Diabetes

Diabetes mellitus is often associated with decreased healing of open wounds and increased susceptibility to infection. Many factors, including peripheral vascular disease, neuropathy, and poor leukocyte function, contribute to poor wound healing in diabetic patients. The dominant mechanism is tissue ischemia caused by microvascular disease.

■ Hematocrit

There are contradictory data regarding the effect of anemia on wound healing. Some researchers have reported a corresponding decrease in wound tensile strength with anemia; others have suggested no change as long as euvolemia is maintained.

■ Nutrition

Animal models simulating malnutrition demonstrate delayed tensile strength of wounds that correlates with the degree of starvation. The effect is particularly severe when starvation occurs early in the healing process.

■ Temperature

Wound healing is accelerated at temperatures close to core body temperature, and it is retarded under conditions of hypothermia.

■ Hydration

Wounds heal best in a warm, moist environment. This explains why occlusive wound dressings and grafts hasten epithelial repair.

■ Steroids and Vitamin A

Corticosteroids negatively affect the inflammatory phase of wound healing by inhibiting wound macrophages and consequently fibrogenesis, angiogenesis, and wound contraction. The deleterious effects of corticosteroids on macrophages are reversed by the administration of vitamin A, 25,000 IU by mouth per day or 200,000 IU topically every 8 hours. Vitamin A deficiency is associated with delayed wound healing, and ingestion of vitamin A stimulates collagen deposition.

■ Nonsteroidal Anti-inflammatory Agents (NSAIDs)

Aspirin and ibuprofen have been shown to decrease collagen synthesis. The effect is mediated by prostaglandins and is dose dependent. No data exist demonstrating that NSAIDs delay wound healing, and most surgeons prescribe NSAIDs in the early postoperative period for pain control.

■ Vitamin C

Vitamin C (ascorbic acid) is an essential cofactor in the synthesis of collagen. Vitamin C deficiency (scurvy) leads to decreased wound tensile strength secondary to immature fibroplasia and failure of formation of mature extracellular materials. It is also marked by formation of defective capillaries, causing local hemorrhages. Even healed wounds deprived of vitamin C lose tensile strength, evidence of the high turnover of collagen over time. As is true for most dietary supplements, excessive intake does not lead to supranormal healing.

■ Vitamin E

Vitamin E has been incorporated into many over-the-counter salves applied to wounds by patients. The evidence to support this practice is entirely anecdotal. In fact, large doses of vitamin E have been found to inhibit wound healing. However, massage and pressure have been shown to flatten and soften scars over the long term. It is possible that some of the perceived benefit is due to these benefits obtained during the process of application.

■ Zinc

Zinc is an important cofactor for many enzyme systems that are important to wound healing. Zinc deficiency has been clearly demonstrated to impair epithelialization and fibroblastic proliferation. Again, excessive intake of Zinc does not lead to supranormal healing.

■ Chemotherapy

Chemotherapy slows the early stages of wound healing and should be delayed for at least 10 to 14 days after wounding. Chemotherapeutic agents generally decrease fibroblast proliferation and wound contraction, leading to delayed wound healing but not deficient wound healing. Generally, medical oncologists wait 2 to 3 weeks after an operation before beginning chemotherapy.

■ Radiation Therapy

Radiation injury leads to arteriolar fibrosis and impaired oxygen delivery. In addition, there is progressive obliteration of blood vessels in the radiated area over time. Radiation also causes intranuclear and cytoplasmic damage to fibroblasts, limiting their proliferative potential.

■ Infection

Infection occurs when the burden of pathogenic organisms overcomes the body's ability to combat them. For most bacterial pathogens, this threshold is 10^5 organisms per gram of tissue. Infection decreases tissue oxygenation and increases collagenolysis, prolonging the inflammatory phase of wound healing and leading to decreased tensile strength. In the presence of significant infection, leukocyte chemotaxis and migration, phagocytosis, and intercellular killing are decreased. Infection also impairs angiogenesis and epithelialization.

■ Age

Controversy exists as to whether age is an independent risk factor for poor wound healing. Epithelialization appears to be more affected than collagen synthesis. Further research into this question is needed before a definitive ruling can be made.

■ Tissue Trauma

Tissue trauma, whether natural or idiopathic, causes increased tissue necrosis. Rough tissue handling, overzealous cauterization, hematoma, tight sutures, tissue ischemia, and subsequent necrosis extend the period of inflammation and retard wound healing.

Abnormalities of Excessive Wound Healing

Many factors are involved in the formation of an ideal scar. The most important of these are:

1. Accurate alignment of sharply incised, viable tissue parallel to the natural lines of resting skin tension.
2. Closure of the wound without tension on the epidermis and without underlying dead space.
3. Primary healing without complications such as infection or dehiscence. The patient's genetic makeup and the location of the wound on the body are also important factors. Hypertrophic scars, keloids, and widespread scars are abnormalities of excessive wound healing found only in humans. They occur in 5% to 15% of wounds and are seen 5 to 15 times more frequently in nonwhites.

■ Hypertrophic Scars

Hypertrophic scars are abnormalities of excessive wound healing that occur within the boundaries of the original wound. The upper torso and flexor surfaces are the usual sites. Hypertrophy occurs more frequently in younger patients, has equal sex predilection, and occurs in blacks and Asians more than whites. These scars usually develop within the first month after wounding and often subside gradually. Hypertrophic scars improve with pressure garments, silicone sheeting applications, or reexcision and closure. Reexcision and closure is a good option, especially if the conditions of closure can be improved (i.e., infection that affected initial healing has resolved).

■ Keloids

True keloids are uncommon and occur predominantly in blacks with a genetic predisposition for keloid formation. They are more frequent in women than in men and most commonly occur in young adults. A keloid rarely subsides without therapy. The primary difference between a keloid and a hypertrophic scar is a keloid's ability to extend beyond the boundaries of the original wound. It behaves as a benign tumor, invading normal surrounding tissue. Keloids affect the face, earlobes, and anterior chest most commonly. The mechanism is uncertain, but elevated levels of immunoglobulin G within the keloid suggests an autoimmune phenomenon. Endocrinologic factors, both androgens and estrogens, have also been implicated because keloids tend to have accelerated growth during puberty or pregnancy and resolve after menopause.

The treatment of keloids is difficult. Surgical reexcision alone has been associated with higher recurrence rates than reexcision combined with local injection of corticosteroids. For moderately large keloids, the addition of pressure therapy in the form of custom compression wraps and garments helps. Finally, for large, treatment-resistant keloids, the best results are reported with a combination of surgery, corticosteroid injection, and postoperative radiotherapy.

■ Widespread Scars

Widespread scars are the result of prolonged mechanical stresses on a wound during the maturation phase of wound healing. They differ from keloids and hypertrophic scars in that they do not exhibit excess collagen deposition but rather collagen deposition at normal levels over a greater surface area. Widespread scars have no genetic, age, ethnic, or sexual predisposition and usually occur within 6 months of wounding. They form most commonly on the arms, legs, and abdomen in areas under constant or repeated tension. Treatment is reexcision and splinting where possible.

Inherited Abnormalities of Deficient Wound Healing

■ Ehlers-Danlos Syndrome (Cutis Hyperelastica)

Cutis hyperelastica is a rare, usually autosomal-dominant disorder characterized by fragile, hyperelastic, and easily bruised skin, joint hypermobility, and aortic aneurysm. Abnormal molecular cross-linking of collagen leads to poor wound healing. The skin has a low tensile strength and does not hold suture material. The surgeon must clearly distinguish the patient with cutis hyperelastica from the patient with cutis laxa, because elective procedures in patients with cutis hyperelastica are fraught with disaster. There are numerous types of Ehlers-Danlos syndrome, each of which has its own set of dangers for the plastic surgeon.

■ Cutis Laxa

Cutis laxa is a rare skin disorder in which the skin hangs in loose folds due to inadequacy of elastic tissue, especially in the skin, lungs, and aorta. Consequently, patients with cutis laxa present with complaints of premature aging, aortic aneurysmal disease, and pulmonary difficulties. The basic mechanism is a nonfunctioning elastase inhibitor or premature degeneration of elastic fibers. Contrary to patients with Ehlers-Danlos syndrome, patients with cutis laxa have normal wound healing. In the absence of cardiorespiratory compromise, operative correction of prematurely aged skin and excision of redundant tissues has been widely successful.

■ Pseudoxanthoma Elasticum

This autosomal-recessive disease is characterized by increased collagen degradation and deposits of calcium and fat on the elastic fibers. The skin has a pebbled appearance with small yellowish papules, extreme laxity, and no rebound. The skin changes are more pronounced in the axilla, groin, and neck. Patients with the disorder are candidates for surgical procedures to correct their deformities, but wound healing problems caused by calcified cutaneous papules and structurally weakened vessels often preclude maximal results.

Wound Management

■ Techniques of Wound Closure

- **Primary healing (by first intention)**—healing by direct approximation of wound margins.
- **Secondary/spontaneous healing (by secondary intention)**—healing by spontaneous granulation, contraction, and epithelialization.
- **Tertiary healing (by third intention)**—delayed closure after a period of time. Contaminated wounds may be closed after a period of time, during which serial débridement has occurred. The advantage to healing by third intention is that it allows for a brief period of wound cleansing prior to closure, theoretically decreasing the risk for wound infection, decreasing time of closure, and improving appearance.

■ Management of Chronic Wounds

A chronic wound is often defined as a wound that has failed to respond to standard care and remains open at 3 months. Typically the wound size is static, and there is an absence of advancing epithelium. The cause is often multifactorial, with ischemia, infection, immunosuppression, edema, or malnutrition often playing a role. A systemic approach is needed to identify all applicable factors that can be controlled. Wounds should be débrided, and topical as well as systemic antibiotics given for bacterial infection. Arterial revascularization can increase oxygenation in the wound, and elevation or compressive dressings can decrease edema. Nutrition can be optimized, and cessation of tobacco use achieved. Glycemic control is critical for those with diabetes. Definitive closure of a chronic wound can be considered only after systemic processes have been treated.

Pressure Ulcers

A pressure ulcer is any lesion caused by unrelieved pressure, resulting in damage of underlying tissue. Pressure ulcers are caused by prolonged friction, shear, pressure, and nutritional debilitation. Moisture, especially that caused by fecal incontinence, has also been implicated as a risk factor. A grading system is based on the depth of the ulcer (Table 2-2).

The best treatment for pressure ulcers is their prevention. Interventions are designed to decrease the amount of pressure, friction, shear, and moisture and to maximize nutritional status.

■ TABLE 2-2 Grading of Pressure Ulcers	
Stage I	Observable pressure-related alteration of intact skin such as altered skin temperature (warm or cool), consistency (firm or boggy), appearance (indurated or pale), and sensation (pain, itching)
Stage II	Partial-thickness skin loss involving epidermis or dermis. A superficial crater, abrasion, or blister.
Stage III	Full-thickness skin loss involving damage or necrosis of subcutaneous tissue down to, but not through, underlying fascia
Stage IV	Full-thickness skin loss with extensive destruction of underlying structures including muscle, tendon, bone, and supporting structures. Tunneling and sinus tracts may be associated.

This can be accomplished through proper positioning techniques and support surfaces, proper incontinence care and moisture control, and a nutritional program. At-risk patients should be turned every 2 hours while in bed and every hour while in a chair. Once an ulcer has formed, intensity of support for the affected areas must increase. To heal a pressure ulcer, pressure must be relieved. The goal is to increase the surface area over which pressure is applied, thereby decreasing the amount of pressure. This is accomplished by using a variety of specialized beds like the Kinair and Clinitron that use air, gel, sand, and water to dissipate pressure.

Surgical treatment of pressure ulcers begins with débridement, possibly under general anesthesia if the ulcer is large. In addition to sharp débridement, pulse lavage, whirlpool treatments, and enzymatic dressings (Table 2-3) can aid in the development of a healthy wound. Once the wound begins to granulate, it becomes a candidate for various closure techniques ranging from skin grafting, to local flap closure, to free tissue transfer. Unfortunately, pressure ulcers have high recurrence rates even in motivated patients.

Lower Extremity Ulcers

Leg ulcers are the most common type of chronic ulcer. The underlying disease process is usually local tissue ischemia. Once the underlying cause of the local ischemia is identified (e.g., venous insufficiency, arterial insufficiency, diabetic-neuropathic origin) proper treatment can be initiated. Table 2-4 compares the types of lower extremity ulcers: venous stasis ulcers, arterial insufficiency ulcers, and diabetic-neuropathic ulcers.

■ TABLE 2-3 Wound Dressings

Classification	Composition	Indications	Advantages	Examples
Hydrocolloids	Contain hydrophilic colloidal particles in an adhesive mass	Clean partial or full-thickness wounds Stage I–IV decubitus ulcers	Absorbs fluid; encourages granulation; promotes epithelialization	Duoderm Comfeel Intrasite Restore
Foams	Either hydrophilic or hydrophobic nonocclusive; usually polyurethane or gel film coated	Partial-thickness wounds that are highly secreting and require mechanical débridement	Débrides; high absorbancy; water vapor permeable	Cutinova Plus Lyofoam Allevyn
Hydrogels	Water with cross-linked polymer; Regranex contains growth factors	Partial-thickness wounds with minimal exudate; excellent in the lower extremity	Moist; low absorbancy; minimally débrides; decreases pain	Intrasite gel Hydrogel Solosite Regranex
Impregnates	Fine mesh gauze impregnated with either moisturizing, antibacterial, or bactericidal compounds	Partial and full-thickness wounds with minimal to moderate exudate; helps clean up a dirty wound	Nonadherent; promotes reepithelialization; antibacterial action	Aquaphor guaze Adaptic Biobrane Scarlet Red Acticoat
Interactive gels and pastes	Medicine-containing gels	Full-thickness wounds with heavy necrosis	Moist environment; débrides	Accuzyme Iodosorb
Vacuum-assisted closure devices	Sponge under negative pressure	Full-thickness wounds with moderate to heavy exudate	Wisks away exudate; promotes angiogenesis; promotes wound contraction	KCI Vac

TABLE 2-4 Characteristics of Lower Extremity Ulcers

	Venous Insufficiency	Arterial Insufficiency	Diabetic-Neuropathic
History	Obesity; DVT or varicosities; traumatic injury; orthopedic procedures; pain reduced by elevation	Increased pain with activity or elevation; smoking, diabetes, hypertension, hypercholesterolemia, peripheral vascular disease	Diabetes; spinal cord injury; paresthesia of extremities
Location	Medial aspect of lower leg and ankle; superior to medial malleolus	Toe tips; web spaces of foot; areas exposed to pressure or repetetive trauma	Plantar aspect of foot; metatarsal heads; heels; sites of painless trauma
Appearance	Shallow, ruddy, irregularly shaped, surrounded by erythema or brownish skin; warm to touch; granulation tissue frequently at base; extremity edematous	Deep, pale, even wound margins; surrounded by pale, shiny skin; evidence of surrounding hair loss; cool to touch; extremity frequently atrophic	Depth variable; surrounding skin appearance variable; commonly indurated; frequent infection; fissuring and callous formation
Perfusion	Pain worse in dependent positions; peripheral pulses present; capillary refill normal	Intermittent claudication or rest pain; peripheral pulses diminished or absent; delayed capillary refill	Peripheral paresthesias; peripheral pulses present; capillary refill normal
Treatment	Elevation; compression garments; vein ligation and stripping; Unna boot; wound dressings that absorb exudate, maintain moist wound surface (alginate, foam, hydrocolloids)	Revascularization procedures; lifestyle changes (exercise, no tobacco, hydration); aggressive treatment of any infection; keep dry wounds dry; keep open wounds moist (hydrogels, interactive gels and pastes)	Tight glucose control; measures to eliminate trauma; appropriate footwear; aggressive infection control; wound dressings to absorb exudate and keep surface moist

Grafts and Flaps

Gedge D. Rosson, MD

THE RECONSTRUCTIVE LADDER

Wound closure can be achieved with a variety of methods that range from simple to complex. The job of the reconstructive plastic surgeon is to choose an appropriate method of wound closure that maximizes form and function while minimizing morbidity. The concept of the "reconstructive ladder" ranks closure methods from simple to complex (Box 3-1).

It presupposes that choosing the lowest rung on the reconstructive ladder provides for success at the lowest cost, a tenant that is usually true. That stated, sometimes a more complex method of closure, or higher rung, gives the best final result. Each wound is evaluated independently and all reconstructive options are considered to provide a reliable, expedient reconstruction that restores form and function.

■ Definitions

- **Graft**: Tissue transferred from one part of the body to another without its blood supply. Basically, a graft is dead once you harvest it, and it slowly comes back to life as it becomes revascularized (Table 3-1).
- **Flap**: Tissue transferred from one part of the body to another with its blood supply intact. A flap is alive when you harvest it, but all or part may die if the blood supply is compromised or inadequate.
- **Free tissue transfer** ("free flap"): A flap whose blood supply is harvested as a pedicle, transferred to a distant site, then anastomosed to recipient vessels.

GRAFTS

Skin Grafts

Skin grafts have been used for centuries to provide coverage for superficial wounds and act as a barrier to infection and trauma.

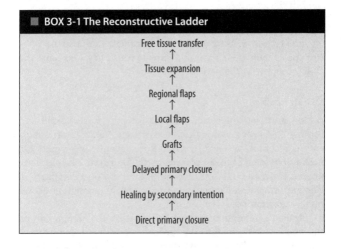

■ BOX 3-1 The Reconstructive Ladder

Free tissue transfer
↑
Tissue expansion
↑
Regional flaps
↑
Local flaps
↑
Grafts
↑
Delayed primary closure
↑
Healing by secondary intention
↑
Direct primary closure

■ TABLE 3-1 Graft Nomenclature

Autograft	Tissue transfer where the same individual is donor and recipient
Isograft	Tissue transfer where donor and recipient are genetically identical, i.e., identical twins
Allograft (aka homograft)	Tissue transfer among members of the same species
Xenograft	Tissue transfer where donor and recipient are of entirely different species

They are harvested as either split-thickness or full-thickness grafts depending on the amount of dermis taken with the graft.

Split-thickness skin grafts (STSGs) contain epidermis and a variable amount of dermis. Their donor sites heal by reepithelialization from epithelial cells located within skin appendages such as hair follicles and sebaceous glands. Due to the absence of epithelial appendages within the graft, STSGs cannot sweat, secrete natural skin oils, or grow hair. Additionally, they contain a variable number of melanocytes, causing altered graft pigmentation. Nerve regeneration in a skin graft occurs over a period of months, with pain sensation returning first and two-point discrimination returning last.

Full-thickness skin grafts (FTSGs) consist of epidermis and the entire dermis. For this reason, an FTSG donor site must be closed by direct primary closure or by a STSG, because the dermal appendages have been removed. Because FTSGs have intact dermal appendages, they can sweat, secrete natural skin oils, and grow hair. They retain a full complement of melanocytes, and thus retain their natural pigmentation. They also have the ability to grow as the patient grows.

■ Graft Healing

A skin graft becomes incorporated into the host wound bed through the process of graft adherence and "take." Graft adherence is accomplished first by a thin fibrin layer between graft and host and later by fibrovascular ingrowth. Skin graft take has three phases: plasmatic imbibition, inosculation, and revascularization. The importance and actual mechanism of each phase is not completely understood.

Plasmatic imbibition occurs for the first 24 to 48 hours. During this phase, grafts gain nutrients through contact with serum on the wound surface. They are considered ischemic and fragile during this phase, and most surgeons go to great lengths to immobilize them during this time. Grafts appear pale and edematous, and may increase their volume by 40% during the imbibition phase.

After 48 hours, **inosculation** begins as capillary buds in the recipient bed contact the graft's microvasculature to establish flow of nutrients between vessels. A fine vascular network is established, and the graft begins to develop a pink hue.

Revascularization, the process by which new vascular channels form to allow actual blood flow between graft and host, begins about 4 days after grafting. Anastomoses form between budding new vessels in the host bed and established vessels in the graft, and these connections provide for nutrition long-term. Early in the revascularization process, which lasts for months, flow is unidirectional from the host to the graft; only as vascular connections mature does the graft develop outflow. For this reason, skin grafts are frequently purplish and swollen in the first weeks to months.

Both STSGs and FTSGs readily form the fibrin bridges necessary for graft adherence. STSGs generally take easier, probably because there is less tissue to be fed by imbibition and inosculation. FTSGs do not take as well and require a much cleaner, more vascular recipient site. FTSGs are more prone to partial take and infection.

■ Contraction

All skin grafts undergo contraction, or shrinkage, and plastic surgeons categorize contraction as primary and secondary. **Primary contraction** occurs immediately upon graft harvest as a result of recoil of dermal elastin fibers. Because FTSGs have more dermis than STSGs, FTSGs undergo more primary contraction. **Secondary contraction** occurs over time as the grafted dermis heals and forms scar. Interestingly, an incomplete dermis undergoes more secondary contraction than a complete dermis; thus, STSGs have more secondary contraction. Secondary contraction can be a pro or a con depending on the anatomic area grafted. For instance, FTSGs are preferred across joints, whereas STSGs are preferred for broad wounds because of their ability to contract the wound over time.

■ Donor Site

Skin can be harvested from any location on the body, but several donor sites for split- and full-thickness skin are favored for cosmetic reasons. Split-thickness skin is most commonly harvested from the thighs and buttocks; less common sites include the back, scalp, breast, and scrotum. Postoperative donor site dressing care is identical to that described for thermal injuries (see Chapter 5).

Full-thickness skin donor sites include areas with excess skin that can be harvested and primarily closed, such as the groin crease, the supraclavicular region, the postauricular area, and the eyelids. Skin from the groin crease tends to be thicker and hair bearing, whereas postauricular and eyelid skin is thin and without hair.

■ Meshing

Meshing, or cutting slits in a graft, is a commonly used method of graft expansion. Meshing allows for greater surface area coverage, greater ease in contouring the graft, and greater egress of fluid. It also helps to minimize the impact of localized bacterial contamination and allows for multiple sites of reepithelialization in the interstices of the graft. Its major disadvantage is the significant amount of secondary healing that must occur, which leads to a "pebbled" appearance. Meshing is most commonly performed in a 1:1.5 ratio, which confers the benefits of meshing while minimizing the pebbled appearance associated with meshed grafts.

■ Complications

The common causes of graft failure are inadequacy of the host wound bed, hematoma, seroma, infection, and sheer forces. Vascularity of the recipient bed plays a vital role—a graft will not take over scar, infected tissue, or dead tissue. Furthermore, it is difficult to obtain graft survival on poorly vascularized structures such as exposed tendon, cortical bone without periosteum, and previously irradiated areas.

Fluid collections such as hematomas, seromas, or lymphoceles block graft take. Meshing an STSG, light pressure dressings, and elevation can help decrease the incidence of fluid collections.

Taking quantitative cultures and testing the wound bed with an allograft prior to definitive autografting can help prevent unexpected infection. Skin grafts will usually take on wound beds with less than 10^5 colonies/mm^3 of bacteria. If an allograft takes without evidence of infection, then an autograft can be expected to take. In the face of infection or colonization, frequent débridement, either sharp or in the form of moist dressing changes, can help minimize graft loss.

Sheering disrupts all three phases of graft take. Efforts to minimize sheer forces include bulky dressings, immobilization of the affected body part, and bedrest.

Nerve Grafts

Nerve grafts are used to reconstruct peripheral nerves when two ends of a severed nerve do not approximate without tension. A nerve graft acts as a guide for distal and proximal ends to meet. The challenge of nerve grafts is proper alignment of sensory and motor fibers because within a given nerve, there are many fascicles, some containing sensory axons, some containing motor axons. After inset, nerve grafts undergo wallerian degeneration similar to the distal segment of an injured native nerve. What remains of the graft is a myelin sheath with Schwann's cells that acts as a biologic conduit for regenerating axons. For a short-segment nerve gap, a prosthetic, hollow neurotube can be substituted. Vein grafts have also been used for short-segment gaps.

The most common nerve graft donor sites are the sural nerve, forearm cutaneous sensory nerves, and greater auricular nerve. Nerve grafts are commonly used in posttraumatic reconstruction of the ulnar nerve in the forearm and reconstruction of the facial nerve to correct facial paralysis. Recovery of nerve function takes months, and results are highly variable. Progress can be monitored by physical examination, electromyography, and sensory testing.

Cartilage Grafts

Cartilage grafts are used for nasal reconstruction, ear reconstruction, and joint reconstruction. Characteristics of cartilage that make it a useful graft are its low nutritional requirements and its viscoelastic properties, which give it "memory." Its low nutritional requirements allow it to survive in poorly vascularized areas with minimal resorption, leading to high long-term success rates. Its ability to retain its shape, or memory, provides a long-lasting result. Reliable cartilage donor sites include the nasal septum, conchal bowl ear cartilage, and rib cartilage. Cartilage for rhinoplasty or nasal reconstruction is usually taken from the nasal septum or the conchal bowl. Cartilage for ear reconstruction is usually taken from the rib.

Bone Grafts

Bone grafts are used to provide rigid, bony reconstruction, and are typically used to fill gaps less than 7 cm in length. The graft can be harvested as cortical, cancellous, or corticocancellous bone, and the method of harvest determines long-term characteristics. After harvest and separation from its native blood supply, grafted bone undergoes necrosis, because only osteocytes on the surface receive nutrients and survive. The remainder of the graft is repopulated by recipient mesenchymal stem cells and blood vessels. Osteoclasts scavenge dead bone, increasing graft porosity and weakening the graft initially. Over time, new osteoblasts invade the graft to deposit new bone. The strength of cortical and cancellous grafts varies with time. Cancellous grafts are structurally weaker at the outset, but are completely replaced by living bone and thus ultimately are stronger. Cortical grafts are stronger initially owing to their preformed cortex, but are never completely replaced by new, living bone and are thus weaker in the long-run. Depending on the location and size, bone grafts reach maturity in 1 to 2 months.

Interestingly, stress also plays a role in maintaining bone graft strength over time. Bone grafts in areas without stress are weaker than those in areas of stress. Preservation of periosteum may also increase graft strength because there is inclusion of increased numbers of osteocytes.

Depending on the amount and shape of bone desired, bone graft can be harvested from the distal radius, the outer table of the calvarium, the ribs, or the iliac crest. (Note: Some plastic surgeons still misuse the term *vascularized bone graft* to refer to a segment of bone harvested along with its vascular supply. Technically, a bone graft taken with its vascular supply is correctly termed a bone flap.)

Tendon Grafts

Tendon grafts are useful for functional upper extremity tendon reconstructions, for lower extremity tendon reconstructions, and as static slings to camouflage facial palsy. Healing of tendon grafts is determined by normal wound healing mechanisms as well as extrinsic forces acting on the tendon. The most commonly harvested tendons are the palmaris longus and the plantaris.

Fat Grafts

Fat grafts are used to correct contour irregularities in soft tissues and for aesthetic augmentation, especially of the lips and cheeks. Lipocytes can be harvested by suction-assisted lipectomy to provide either macrografts or micrografts, or by direct excision either with or without an accompanying dermal graft. The results of fat grafting are quite variable based on technique, vascularity of the recipient bed, quality of the donor fat, and the skill and experience of the surgeon. In general, the success rate of fat grafts is not as good as other tissue grafting, and long-term correction and augmentation are achieved only about half the time.

Composite Grafts

Composite grafts incorporate two or more tissue types into a single graft. Their survival depends on the variable metabolic needs of their component parts as well as access of the components to recipient site blood supply. Examples of composite grafts include chondrocutaneous grafts from the ear to reconstruct the nose and dermofascial fat grafts to various areas of the face for facial rejuvenation.

FLAPS

Angiosomes

Angiosomes are regions of skin and underlying deep tissue supplied by a source artery. These perforators can either be direct, going from the source vessel straight to the skin, or indirect, supplying an underlying muscle primarily and an overlying skin region secondarily. Angiosomes are the vascular equivalent of the neurologic concept of the dermatome, and they are the basis for all flaps that contain skin. Understanding the body's angiosomes has been critical to the development of flaps, and in turn has revolutionized soft tissue reconstruction.

Flap Classification

■ Method of Transfer

Flap transfer is described as local or distant based on whether the flap is adjacent to the recipient bed. Local flaps are adjacent to their recipient bed and either advance or pivot. Examples of advancement flaps include the "V to Y" and the rectangular advancement flap (see Chapter 1). Examples of pivot flaps include rotation, transposition, and island flaps (see Chapter 1).

Distant flaps are not adjacent to their recipient bed and include the cross-leg flap, groin flaps to the hand, and Tagliocozzi's arm flap to the nose. Microvascular free tissue transfers are also examples of distant flaps.

■ Blood Supply

Random pattern flaps lack a known vascular supply, and are fed by the subdermal and dermal plexus, which usually supports a 1:2 or 1:3 width to length ratio. Slightly longer random flaps can survive in the head and neck, due to the greater density of perforating vessels and greater density of the dermal plexus. Random pattern flaps below the clavicles are designed with a 1:2 width to length ratio to provide reliable vascularity to the tip of the flap.

Arterial, or **axial**, skin flaps have a named artery as the blood supply to the flap. This allows for a greater length to width ratio. Examples include the groin flap and the lateral arm flap. Axial flaps can be supplied by a musculocutaneous artery or a septocutaneous artery as the main source. Musculocutaneous axial flaps (such as the pedicled transverse rectus abdominis myocutaneous [TRAM] flap, see Chapter 7) are well vascularized because the muscle is included in the flap and the overlying skin is supplied by musculocutaneous perforators. Septocutaneous artery flaps are supplied by a named vessel that runs in the deep tissues and sends perforators through the facial or septal attachments to the overlying soft tissues of the flap (such as the radial forearm flap).

■ Flap Composition

Flaps can also be classified according to the tissues that comprise them. Examples include adipocutaneous, fasciocutaneous, muscular, myocutaneous, osteocutaneous, or any combination of the above. A fibular free flap for mandibular reconstruction containing bone, a cuff of muscle, and the overlying skin paddle would be classified as an osteomyocutaneous free flap.

Fasciocutaneous Flaps

A fasciocutaneous flap is a paddle of skin supplied by the vascular plexus of the underlying fascia. The fascia itself is supplied by branches of arteries running in the septae between muscle bellies. The radial forearm flap is a classic example of a fasciocutaneous flap used in head and neck reconstruction, penile reconstruction, and even esophageal reconstruction. Fasciocutaneous flaps can be harvested and inset with a sensory nerve to provide a sensate reconstruction.

The evolution of soft tissue reconstruction is toward a more versatile flap with less donor site morbidity. With that in mind, microsurgeons have begun to leave behind the fascia underlying fasciocutaneous flaps to create an adipocutaneous flap that is more pliable and leaves less of a donor site defect. For example, the anterolateral thigh flap can be harvested with or without the deep fascia of the thigh.

Muscle Flaps and Myocutaneous Flaps

Myocutaneous flaps are compound flaps composed of the muscle, its fascia, and the overlying subcutaneous fat and skin. They are supplied by the dominant vascular pedicle to the muscle. From the muscle, multiple perforating vessels supply the skin. According to Mathes and Nahai, muscles can be classified into five types based on vascular supply. The vascular supply determines how a muscle flap is harvested and what portion of the muscle can be counted on if based on a single pedicle. Any muscle that can be supplied solely by its dominant pedicle is a useful muscle flap. The most common type of muscle found in the body is a type 2 muscle. Type 4 muscles are less useful as muscle flaps due to their segmental blood supply.

Muscle flaps have excellent blood flow, and reportedly have better success in infected and irradiated wounds. They are malleable, fitting into crevasses better than an adipofascial flap. Muscle flaps are reliable due to fairly constant vascular anatomy, and they can be innervated for a functional reconstruction. Common examples of muscle flaps uses include the TRAM flap for breast reconstruction, the gracilis flap for groin wound coverage, the soleus flap for coverage of pretibial wounds, and the pectoralis flap for treatment of sternal osteomyelitis.

The Delay Phenomenon

Flap delay involves ligation of some of the vessels supplying a flap in order to force it to gain its nutrition from elsewhere. Ligation causes a reorganization of vascular flow in a flap to maximize flow to the distalmost segment. The purpose of delaying a flap is to increase the amount of distal flap that ultimately survives after harvest. Maximum effect is seen approximately 7 to 14 days after the delay procedure. The benefits of recruiting extra tissue by flap delay must be weighed against the cost of adding another procedure and time to a reconstruction.

A good example of the delay phenomenon is the pedicled TRAM flap, which is based on the superior epigastric artery, the rectus muscle's nondominant pedicle. Ligation of the rectus muscle's dominant pedicle, the deep inferior epigastric artery,

10 days prior to flap harvest gives the muscle time to adjust to its new vascular supply prior to placing the flap on the chest wall for breast reconstruction. Some researchers claim greater success with the pedicled TRAM flap after delay.

Microvascular Free Tissue Transfer

The first free flap was described in a dog study in 1963 by Goldwyn when he elevated a groin flap, divided the pedicle, and then reattached it using microvascular techniques. The first human microvascular free flap was performed by Buncke in 1972 when he transferred an omental flap to the superficial temporal vessels for scalp reconstruction. Since that time, nearly every angiosome has been described as a donor for free tissue transfer. Like their pedicled cousins, free tissue transfers are classified by their composite tissues as adipocutaneous, fasciocutaneous, muscular, myocutaneous, and osteocutaneous free flaps. Although several free flap donor sites are popular due to reliability, diameter and length of the nutrient artery (pedicle), and ease of harvest, no single free flap is ideal for all situations. Certain free flaps are valuable for specific reconstructions, such as the fibula free flap for mandibular reconstruction, the free TRAM flap for breast reconstruction, and the innervated free gracilis for facial reanimation.

■ Perforator Flaps

As stated earlier, the evolution of soft tissue reconstruction is toward a more versatile flap with less donor site morbidity. A perforator flap is an adipocutaneous free flap based on a pedicle that perforates, or bores through, either a muscle or muscular septum. A skin flap that is supplied by a muscle perforator is called a **musculocutaneous perforator flap**. A skin flap that is supplied by a septal perforator is called a **septocutaneous perforator flap**. A perforator flap is named after the nutrient artery or vessels that supply it, and not after the underlying muscle (i.e., deep inferior epigastric perforator [DIEP] flap, rather than the transverse rectus abdominus musculocutaneous perforator [TRAMP] flap). If there is a potential to harvest multiple perforator flaps from one vessel, the name of each flap should be based on its anatomic region or muscle (i.e., anterolateral thigh [ALT] flap). Perforator flaps allow for harvest of thinner, less bulky flaps with decreased donor site morbidity, because the underlying muscle or fascia is left in place.

Clinical examples of perforator flaps include the DIEP flap and the superior gluteal artery perforator (SGAP) flap, both commonly used for breast reconstruction, and the ALT flap, commonly used in head and neck reconstruction.

■ Anticoagulation

Various anticoagulant medications have been used both intraoperatively and postoperatively to enhance blood flow in microvascular free tissue transfer. Aspirin, subcutaneous heparin, intravenous heparin, dextran, low-molecular-weight heparin, leech therapy, Hespan, streptokinase, and urokinase have all been tested, and none has demonstrated an ability to alter free flap failure rates. That stated, most microsurgeons use some form of medicinal anticoagulation for their free flaps. Aspirin and heparin are used most frequently, either separately or in combination.

■ Free Flap Monitoring

It is important to monitor flap perfusion and viability in the acute postoperative period so that anastomotic failure can be fixed before a flap dies. Numerous machines have been invented to assist with this process, including laser Doppler flowmeters, differential thermometers, fluorescein dye injection, radioisotope staining, and electromagnetic flowmeters. None has proven more effective than serial physical examination by an experienced surgeon. Flap surgeons evaluate flap color, capillary refill, tissue turgor, and Doppler signal. Healthy flaps are neither pale nor purple, but rather have a pink color. Capillary refill is around 2 seconds, not too brisk or too sluggish, which would indicate venous engorgement or arterial insufficiency. The Doppler signal should be biphasic, and without a forceful "water hammer" sound. Taken together, these signs allow experienced flap surgeons to monitor their results without the need for expensive equipment.

TISSUE EXPANSION

Tissue expansion is a mechanical process that increases the surface area of local tissue available for reconstructive procedures. Silicone balloons are implanted below the skin surface and inflated over time to "expand" the overlying soft tissue (Figure 3-1). Forces of expansion induce an increase in epidermal mitosis and tissue recruitment. Tissue expansion can be used alone or as an adjunct to more complicated reconstructions; it is a reliable technique that preserves hair and sensibility of tissues, while providing a good color and texture match.

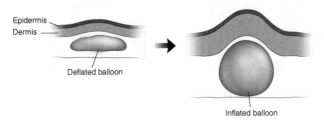

Epidermis
Dermis

Deflated balloon

Inflated balloon

Figure 3-1 • Tissue expansion.

Tissue expansion induces interesting physiologic and histologic changes in affected tissues. The epidermis thickens, while
dermis, fat, and muscle thin. Muscle does not lose the ability to
contract; fat thinning and atrophy is permanent. Importantly, tissues are not merely stretched—there is a true net gain of tissue.
Histologically, the epidermis displays cellular hyperplasia, and
the basilar layer has an increased rate of mitosis. Dermal elastic
fibers stretch and may fracture, and muscle sarcomeres and mito-
chondria undergo configurational changes. Vascularity increases
dramatically, particularly at the junction of the capsule and
normal surrounding tissue. Two important mechanical properties
of viscoelastic materials come into play during the acute inflation
of tissue expanders: creep and stress-relaxation. **Creep** is the
time-dependent deformation of a material to a constantly applied
force. **Stress-relaxation** is the principle that the amount of force
required to stretch a material to a constant length will decrease
over time.

Once tissue expanders are placed, filling begins in 2 or
3 weeks, and they are filled at a rate commensurate with tissue
creep and stress relaxation. They are filled to the point of causing
pain, indicating tissue ischemia, with careful monitoring of tissues for signs of necrosis and potential extrusion of silicone prostheses.

Tissue expanders are produced in a variety of shapes and sizes
for use over the entire body. Common uses include breast reconstruction, defects on the abdomen and chest, scalp reconstruction,
and cervicofacial flap reconstruction. They are used increasingly in
the subacute treatment of thermal injuries, as well. Complications
include infection, prosthetic extrusion, and pain.

Chapter

4

Skin and Soft Tissue

Michele Ann Manahan, MD

Skin is the barrier to dehydration and environmental pathogens, a regulator of body temperature via sweat glands and a rich vascular supply, a key contact point for the body's immune system, and a highly specialized sensory organ. The outer epidermis and the inner dermis are separated by a basement membrane. The epidermis consists mostly of stratified squamous epithelium composed of keratinocytes, but also contains specialized sensory end organs called Merkel's cells, pigment-producing melanocytes, and immunologically oriented Langerhans' cells. The relatively acellular dermis is the strength layer of the skin and is commonly divided into the superficial "papillary" dermis and deep "reticular" dermis. It is largely composed of collagens, elastin, and ground substance but also contains fibroblasts, histiocytes, and agents of the immune system. The dermis supports pilosebaceous units that produce oil and hair, eccrine sweat glands, apocrine sweat glands, nerves, blood vessels (subdermal plexus and papillary dermal plexus), and lymphatics (Figure 4-1).

SKIN CANCER

Basal Cell Carcinoma

■ Epidemiology and Risk Factors

Skin cancer is the most common cancer in the United States, with about 800,000 new cases diagnosed yearly. Basal cell carcinoma (BCC) is the most common variety, accounting for over 75% of cases. Sun exposure is the major risk factor, although prior radiation and immunosuppression also increase the risk. Various inherited disorders like xeroderma pigmentosum and albinism are risk factors for the development of BCC. The typical patient with BCC is a man in his fifth to seventh decade of life with a history of sun exposure and fair skin that burns easily. Over 90% of BCC occurs on the head and neck, with about one fourth arising on the nose.

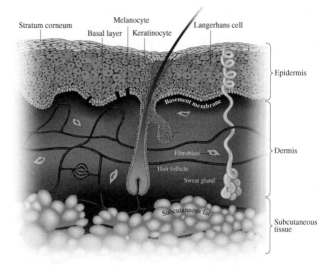

Figure 4-1 • Cross-section of the skin.

■ Diagnosis

Classically, BCCs present as scaly ulcers with rolled edges, so-called "rodent ulcers" because of their appearance. Suspicious lesions are examined via biopsy either via an excisional biopsy to completely eradicate the tumor or via an incisional biopsy.

There are three morphologic types: noduloulcerative, superficial, and sclerosing. **Noduloulcerative** basal cell carcinoma, the most common, is a pearly papule with overlying telangiectasias. **Superficial** BCC is a red, scaly lesion similar to squamous cell carcinoma, and there are often multiple lesions. **Sclerosing** BCC is the type most likely to recur and presents as a yellow-white patch with ill-defined borders, resembling a scar.

■ Treatment

Basal cell carcinomas rarely metastasize, but their growth can lead to extensive destruction of adjacent structures. Small lesions (less than 1 cm) are often treated by electrodesiccation, cryotherapy, or curettage. Larger lesions merit surgical resection with histologic confirmation of negative margins. Typically, excisions are planned with 2- to 4-mm margins. Frozen sections may be sent from the specimen to prove that the margins of resection are free of tumor.

In aesthetically sensitive areas, Mohs' micrographic surgery may be preferred. This involves serial excision of paper thin slices of tissue with immediate microscopic examination of frozen sections to determine when negative margins have been achieved. Local radiotherapy is reserved for cases where surgery is not an option.

■ Prognosis

Most cases are treatable, and cure rates are high. However, follow-up is indicated every 6 months for 5 years following diagnosis and treatment. Recurrence is a persistent problem, largely due to inaccurate assessment of tumor borders leading to inadequate resection. Recurrence is more common in the central face, ear, and forehead. Mohs' micrographic surgery is the treatment of choice for recurrent lesions.

Squamous Cell Carcinoma

■ Epidemiology and Risk Factors

Squamous cell carcinoma (SCC) of the skin is one fourth as prevalent as BCC. Risk factors include exposure to sun, radiotherapy, human papilloma virus, chronic inflammation (ulceration, sinus tracts, osteomyelitis, burns), immunosuppression, tar, psoralens, atmospheric pollution, arsenic, and nitrogen mustard. Dermatoses, hidradenitis suppurativa, and lupus erythematosus may predispose to squamous cell carcinoma by causing chronic wounds. Actinic (solar) keratoses and *in situ* lesions (Bowen's disease or erythroplasia of Queyrat when involving mucous membranes such as the anus, mouth, or genitalia) are red, scaly, maculopapular precursors.

■ Diagnosis

Squamous cell carcinomas usually arise in areas of sun-damaged skin. They begin as nodules that may ulcerate. Induration and necrosis are more prominent with SCC than with BCC. As with BCC, incisional or shave biopsy is needed for diagnosis, and it usually demonstrates irregular masses of proliferating atypical keratinocytes invading the dermis.

■ Treatment

Surgical excision with 1-cm margins and histologic confirmation of complete resection is usually the treatment of choice. As with basal cell carcinoma, Mohs' micrographic surgery may be preferred for tumors occurring in cosmetically sensitive areas. Regional lymphadenectomy is indicated for palpable nodal disease as well as clinically negative (nonpalpable) nodal basins in the setting of SCCs in areas of chronic inflammation. As with BCC, radiation is reserved for patients who are poor operative candidates or who refuse surgery. Topical 5-fluorouracil is an excellent therapy for premalignant lesions associated with SCC, such actinic keratoses, but it is not recommended for the primary treatment of SCC.

■ Prognosis

Like BCCs, SCCs may lead to widespread surrounding tissue destruction. However, these tumors also carry a significant risk for metastasis. Tumor thickness and location are important prognostic indicators. Lesions that are thicker than 4 mm and those on the ear, nostril, scalp, and extremities are prone to local recurrence and metastasis. Lesions thicker than 10 mm and those occurring in areas of chronic inflammation (Marjolin's ulcer), Bowen's disease, or erythroplasia of Queyrat tend to metastasize more frequently. When the primary tumor is in an extremity, the presence of nodal disease carries a dismal prognosis, with only a 35% 5-year survival rate. Recurrence is also more common in poorly differentiated tumors and those with perineural invasion. Reexcision is the optimal treatment for recurrent disease. Most patients survive this disease, and follow-up should occur every 3 months for several years following diagnosis and treatment. Follow-up intervals may eventually be lengthened to 6 months.

Melanoma

■ Epidemiology and Risk Factors

The incidence of melanoma is around 40,000 cases per year in the United States and is increasing by 5% per year. The reason for this acute increase is uncertain and cannot be attributed to sun exposure alone. Melanoma is the leading cause of skin cancer deaths in the United States, accounting for about 1% of all cancer deaths.

Risk factors for the development of melanoma include actinic exposure (especially blistering sunburns during childhood), fair hair and skin, blue eyes, freckling with sun exposure, Northern European ancestry, presence of multiple moles, relatives with melanoma, immunosuppression, and genetic conditions such as the autosomal-dominant atypical mole syndrome (dysplastic nevus syndrome). Melanomas are most common on the head and neck. Men have a propensity for trunk melanomas; women have a propensity for lower extremity melanomas.

Public awareness through the mass media and screening programs has improved early detection of melanoma. Other means of prevention include wearing sunscreen and protective clothing to limit UV radiation, and self-awareness of the presence of atypical moles.

■ Clinical Manifestations

The hallmarks of malignant melanoma are **A**symmetry, **B**order irregularity, **C**olor variegation, and large **D**iameter (>6 mm). Generally, melanomas are thought of as going through two growth phases: radial and vertical. The radial growth phase is a period when malignant melanocytes are contained within the epidermis and papillary dermis and cell growth occurs laterally. There is little concern of metastasis during this phase. The vertical growth phase, in contrast, is characterized by rapid invasion of deeper structures, signaling a more aggressive tumor with metastatic potential. Most histologic types of melanoma go through a radial growth phase before going into a vertical growth phase. The exception is nodular melanoma, which goes directly to a vertical growth phase and is therefore thought of as highly invasive. The four histologic types of melanoma are reviewed in Table 4-1.

■ Differential Diagnosis

The differential diagnosis of pigmented lesions includes many benign and premalignant lesions. A **lentigo** is a generic term for a pigmented, macular (flat) lesion with a reticular pattern. A simple lentigo is indistinguishable from a junctional nevus, whereas a solar lentigo is lighter and commonly known as a liver spot. Benign nevi include junctional nevi, compound nevi, and blue nevi. Melanoma precursors, which by definition have atypical melanocytes with a potential for malignant degeneration, include the dysplastic nevus, melanoma *in situ* (clinically identical to the dysplastic nevus), and lentigo maligna (otherwise known as Hutchinson's freckle). Congenital nevi (1% incidence) are often larger and frequently contain hair. Giant congenital nevi are cosmetically disfiguring and possess a 5% risk for progression to melanoma.

■ Diagnosis

The diagnosis of melanoma is made by full-thickness biopsy of any suspicious lesion. There are three acceptable biopsy techniques for diagnosing melanoma: excisional, incisional, and punch.

- An excisional biopsy is indicated for small lesions.
- An incisional biopsy may be performed in areas where maximal skin preservation is essential.
- A punch biopsy is indicated for large lesions, and must be performed on the most raised area. *A shave biopsy, electrocoagulation, or electrodesiccation should NEVER be performed for pigmented lesions since these methods obliterate information regarding thickness, which is essential for determining prognosis and therapy.*

TABLE 4-1 Characteristics of Histological Types of Melanoma

Type of Melanoma	Proportion of Cases	Mean Age at Diagnosis (yr)	Affected Sites	Clinical Features
Superficial Spreading	70%	50's	Entire body; torso; legs in females	Raised border; can be brown, black, blue, gray, amelanotic; horizontal growth
Nodular	15%	40's	Entire body (most commonly on head and neck, back)	Mostly vertical growth; nodular brown to black lesion; can arise from normal skin or a mole
Acral Lentiginous	10%	60's	Soles, palms, mucous membranes, subungual	Flat with irregular border; brown or black; early intradermal phase makes it more aggressive because of late diagnosis
Lentigo Maligna	5%	70's	Nose, cheeks, temples	Highly irregular borders; regression more common; variation in pigment pattern

In addition to examination of tissue, a workup of melanoma includes history and physical examination (including skin, all palpable lymph node groups, neurologic function), chest x-ray, and liver function tests (including LDH). Those patients with abnormal findings need further imaging studies.

■ Clinical Staging

Clinical staging is used to direct therapy and to prognosticate. Although many aspects of the primary tumor affect prognosis, the most important factors are the **thickness of the lesion** and the **presence of ulceration**. Thickness may be described by two methods: Clark's levels and Breslow thickness. Breslow thickness describes absolute tumor thickness (in millimeters) and is the primary determinant of prognosis. Breslow thickness has been used to coin the terms most often to describe melanoma's as thin (<1 mm), intermediate thickness (1–4 mm), and thick (>4 mm). Clark's level is a description of the anatomic depth of invasion, which correlates loosely with thickness (Table 4-2).

Apart from characteristics of the primary tumor, lymph node status and presence of distant metastasis are also primary determinants of prognosis. The American Joint Committee on Cancer has developed a staging system based on the Tumor, Node, Metastasis (TNM) system that is widely used today (Table 4-3).

■ Treatment

There are three considerations in the treatment of melanoma: (1) eradication of the primary tumor, (2) treatment of regional lymph nodes, and (3) treatment of metastatic disease. Increasing tumor thickness requires wider margins of excision. Current recommendations for margins of excision are in Table 4-4. Tumors on the digits may require amputation. Subungual melanoma requires partial amputation of the involved digit.

Palpable nodal disease requires regional lymphadenectomy. Nonpalpable lymph nodes with intermediate thickness (1–4 mm thick) melanomas may be sampled by sentinel lymph node biopsy. Sentinel lymph node biopsy is based on the observation

■ TABLE 4-2 Clark's Levels of Invasion

Level	Tissue Invaded
I	Epidermis only
II	Into papillary dermis
III	Papillary-reticular junction
IV	Into reticular dermis
V	Into subcutaneous tissue

■ TABLE 4-3 AJCC Staging System for Melanoma

TNM	Criteria
T1	Tumor ≤1.0 mm
T2	Tumor 1.1–2.0 mm
T3	Tumor 2.1–4.0 mm
T4	Tumor >4.0 mm
Ta	No ulceration
Tb	Ulceration
N1	1 positive node
N2	2–3 positive nodes
N3	≥4 positive nodes, intransit or satellite lesions
Na	Microscopic disease
Nb	Macroscopic disease
M1a	Metastases to skin, subcutaeous tissue, lymph nodes
M1b	Metastases to lung
M1c	All other metastases, any mets with elevated LDH

Stage	T	N	M
I	T1a&b;T2a	N_0	M_0
II	T2b to T4b	N_0	M_0
III	any T	any N	M_0
IV	any T	any N	M_1

■ TABLE 4-4 Surgical Margins for Excision Melanoma

Tumor Thickness (mm)	Surgical Margin (cm)
In situ	0.5
<1.0	1
1–2	1–2
2–4	2
>4	2–4

that melanoma cells will metastasize first to the group of lymph nodes that is immediately upstream from the affected region about 98% of the time. Thus, if a surgeon maps out that group of lymph nodes by using either a radioactive tracer or a colored dye, he may find that group of lymph nodes and resect them. If the sentinel lymph nodes are negative for tumor, the patient is spared a lymphadenectomy; if the nodes are positive, a lymphadenectomy is performed. Thus, sentinel lymph node biopsy is a method of sparing some patients with intermediate-thickness melanoma a regional lymphadenectomy. The efficacy of elective lymphadenectomy remains a hotly debated topic.

Melanoma has a tendency to recur many years after initial diagnosis; therefore, follow-up should be lifelong. Suspected recurrences should be worked up with a chest x-ray and liver function tests. Recurrences may be treated by wide local excision (solitary lesions of the skin, subcutaneous tissue, liver, lung, or brain) with or without regional lymphadenectomy, or adjuvant methods such as radiotherapy, chemotherapy, isolated limb perfusion, and immunotherapy. Adjuvant therapies are usually reserved for patients who are not surgical candidates.

■ Prognosis

Overall 5-year survival for melanoma is 89%. Five-year survival for those who present with local, regional, and distant disease is 96%, 61%, and 12%, respectively. The skin, subcutaneous tissue, and lymph nodes are the most common sites of recurrence and metastasis. The lungs, liver, bone, brain, and intestines, respectively, are the most common visceral organs involved in metastatic melanoma. Average survival after diagnosis of metastases is 6 months. Death from melanoma occurs most often due to respiratory failure secondary to pulmonary metastases followed by brain metastases.

HEMANGIOMAS AND VASCULAR MALFORMATIONS

Hemangiomas

■ Epidemiology

Hemangiomas are the most common neoplasm noted during infancy. They arise in early infancy and grow rapidly by endothelial proliferation. They then undergo gradual, spontaneous involution throughout childhood in 90% of cases. They affect about 1% of children at birth and up to 10% of children by age 1 year, most commonly white females.

■ Clinical Manifestations

The initial lesion is a patch of erythema, hypopigmentation, or telangiectasias with pale halos known as "herald spots." It evolves to an irregular, red, spongy mass that can be multiple. The lesion initially appears to be more superficial (capillary) and progresses to a deeper lesion (cavernous). Signs of involution include central pallor, less intense color, and shrinkage.

■ Diagnosis

The main diagnostic dilemma is differentiating between hemangiomas and vascular malformations. Hemangioma growth exceeds the rate of growth of the child. The color changes as it grows. The "doughy" consistency is also characteristic, and no skeletal changes occur. CT or MRI can aid in diagnosis and demonstrate well-circumscribed homogeneous lesions. In extreme cases, arteriography may be useful. The diagnostic workup also includes examination for visceral hemangiomas and underlying structural abnormalities of the brain, spinal cord, or vasculature.

■ Treatment

Treatment usually consists of watchful waiting. Immunosuppressants, laser therapy, embolization, or surgical excision is necessary for lesions that ulcerate, bleed, or become infected. Hemangiomas that affect vision, hearing, feeding, breathing, or urination must also be excised. Thrombocytopenia and high output cardiac failure are infrequent complications. Surgical excision is also indicated for easily removable facial lesions in children preparing to enter school and those lesions remaining into adolescence.

Vascular Malformations

■ Epidemiology and Clinical Manifestations

Vascular malformations begin with faulty embryogenesis. These nonneoplastic lesions do not proliferate or invade surrounding tissues. Unlike hemangiomas, they grow as the body grows and change appearance with blood pressure fluctuations. The most common venous malformation is the superficial lower extremity varicosity, affecting 1% to 4% of individuals. Arteriovenous malformations present as warm, discolored subcutaneous masses with a palpable thrill and bruit by auscultation. They can cause pain, ulceration, bleeding, congestive heart failure, and destruction of surrounding structures. Port-wine stain (nevus flammeus), another variant, is composed of intradermal capillaries, is present at birth, and does not regress. It may present as a red macule, often in the distribution of the trigeminal nerve, making it aesthetically significant. Most are sporadic, but it may be seen in combination with leptomeningeal angiomas, epilepsy, and glaucoma (Sturge-Weber syndrome). Arterial malformations are usually asymptomatic and are diagnosed during adulthood.

■ Diagnosis

History, physical examination, imaging techniques (ultrasound, CT, or MRI), and histopathologic examination are often necessary to arrive at a diagnosis. MRI has emerged as the imaging modality of choice for diagnosing vascular malformations.

■ Treatment

Venous malformations may be treated with sclerosis, laser therapy, or resection. The complications of arteriovenous malformations often require angiographic embolization or surgical resection; however, the treatment varies with location. Laser therapy is the treatment of choice for port-wine stains.

INFECTIONS

Hidradenitis Suppurativa

Hidradenitis suppurativa is a bacterial infection of the apocrine sweat glands. It presents as inflammation, abscesses, and draining sinus tracts in the groin and axilla. Hidradenitis tends to be chronic and may be treated with excision of affected areas. However, surgery for an acute flare is not indicated unless presence of a necrotizing infection is suspected. These are routinely managed with medical therapies like warm compresses, antistaphylococcal antibiotics, and meticulous hygiene.

Cutaneous Cysts

Pilonidal cysts are infected pilosebaceous units. They usually occur in young, moderately obese, hirsute males. Frequently, they present as an indurated, painful mass above the anus in the gluteal fold. Acute infections should be incised and drained. If left untreated, a sinus tract may form and epithelialize. Obliteration of the sinus tract via curettage, excision and primary closure, marsupialization, or flap coverage is the definitive treatment.

Other cutaneous cysts that present similarly to pilonidal cysts but in different locations are epidermal inclusion cysts, trichilemmal cysts, and dermoid cysts. These firm nodules contain a creamy exudate of sloughed epithelial cells and may rupture, become inflamed, or form an abscess. Surgical excision is the definitive therapy.

Folliculitis

Folliculitis, cellulitis of a hair follicle, can progress to become a furuncle, or abscess of the hair follicle. When a furuncle spreads within the deep tissues and begins to drain via multiple sinus tracts, it is called a carbuncle. Treatment of these interrelated conditions requires meticulous hygiene, warm soaks, and antistaphylococcal antibiotics. Most carbuncles resolve without surgical débridement, but wide local excision is an option.

Other Cutaneous Conditions

- **Actinomycosis** is a fungal infection that forms abscesses of the jaw and face. They may form fistulas and extend to facial bones and lung apices. Sulfur granules on microscopic examination are diagnostic. These are routinely managed with antibiotics, reserving surgical drainage for extreme cases.
- **Lymphogranuloma venereum** (LGV) is caused by the sexually transmitted, intracellular gram-negative bacterium *Chlamydia trachomatis*. Following resolution of a genital ulcer, large, painful inguinal lymphadenopathy develops and may suppurate. Surgical drainage is avoided because this leads to formation of chronic sinus tracts. Antibiotics (doxycycline or azithromycin) are the treatments of choice.
- **Condylomata** (herpetic warts) are hyperkeratotic papules appearing in clusters on the skin. These lesions are sometimes macerated, secondarily infected, and malodorous. Small lesions are best managed with either curettage and electrodesiccation or liquid nitrogen. Excisional cure is difficult to obtain due to indistinct margins.
- **Staphylococcal scalded skin syndrome** occurs almost exclusively in the pediatric population. Exotoxins produced by staphylococci cause erythema, bullae, and skin denudation. Involvement of the mucous membranes and conjuctiva is not seen.
- **Toxic epidermal necrolysis (TENS) and Stevens-Johnson syndrome (SJS)** are characterized by epidermal slough at the dermal–epidermal junction due to an immunologic reaction. They represent a continuum of disease whose most innocuous form is **erythema multiforme**. Extensive skin loss and mucous membrane involvement merits intensive supportive care and local wound care as in acute thermal injury (see Chapter 5). Intravenous steroids have been associated with increased morbidity and mortality in TENS or SJS.

LYMPHEDEMA

■ Anatomy of the Lymphatic System

The purpose of the lymphatic system is the return of fluid and proteins from the interstitium to the intravascular space. Superficial, valveless lymph channels originate in the epidermis and drain into deeper channels equipped with one-way valves and smooth muscle that aid in peristaltic movement of lymph. The lymphatic fluid then travels into major regional lymph node groups via the subcutaneous collectors or by way of deep lymphatics that run with local neurovascular bundles. Major lymph node groups located at the

> ### ■ BOX 4-1 Causes of Lymphedema
>
> **Primary**
> Congenital (onset at birth)
> Praecox (onset during puberty)
> Tarda (onset in adulthood)
> **Secondary**
> Malignancy
> Surgical disruption of lymphatics—lymph node dissection, groin exploration
> Radiation
> Recurrent cellulitis
> Connective tissue disorders
> Infection (filariasis)
> Contact dermatitis

base of each limb filter lymph and act as an important contact point with the immune system. Major lymph vessels coalesce to form the thoracic duct, which opens into the angle between the left subclavian vein and the left jugular vein.

■ Etiology

Lymphedema is classified as either primary (occurring spontaneously) or secondary (a manifestation of a disease process). Parasitic infection is the leading cause of lymphedema worldwide, most commonly due to filariasis. The leading cause of lymphedema in the United States is malignancy (Box 4-1).

■ Clinical Manifestations

Lymphedema typically presents with nonpitting swelling in an extremity, usually with involvement of the digits. The onset of secondary lymphedema is usually insidious, but may be abrupt following local inflammation from infection or limb injury. Some patients complain of "heaviness" in the affected extremity and limitation in range of motion. With time, the skin becomes dry and firm with fibrosis. All patients should be inspected for signs of cellulitis and treated with antistaphylococcal antibiotics if present. Lymphangitis, which causes a tender macular rash overlying an infected lymphatic must also be ruled out. Rarely, patients with chronic lymphedema develop a secondary malignant lymphangiosarcoma, which appears as a blue-red or purple maculopapular skin lesion.

■ Diagnosis

Diagnosis is based largely on physical examination. Other causes of limb swelling, such as deep venous thrombosis, malignancy, and infection, must be ruled out with the appropriate studies. Imaging modalities that aid physical diagnosis include radionuclide lymphoscintigraphy and lymphangiography (rarely performed). MRI and CT, which provide additional anatomic and nodal detail, may complement lymphoscintigraphy.

■ Treatment

Patients undergoing procedures known to cause lymphedema, like elective lymph node dissection or radiation, may be counseled in preventive measures. These include avoiding blood draws or IV lines in the affected extremity, heavy activity in the affected limb, keeping the limb in a dependent position, wearing tight fitting clothing, and infection. Meticulous hygiene is critical.

The goal of treatment of lymphedema is to control limb swelling since the underlying disease is often uncorrectable. Furthermore, if untreated, lymphedema tends to progress and to inhibit the activities of daily living.

Most lymphedema can be successfully treated with conservative, nonoperative therapies. Nonsurgical treatments include exercise, gradient pressure garments, ACE wraps, massage therapy, and external pneumatic compression devices. Most widely used are gradient pressure garments, which generate greater pressure distally than proximally to promote mobilization of edema. Remember that lymphedema is a mechanical problem, and pharmacologic therapies have been of little help. Diuretics are sometimes tried with little benefit, and may promote the development of volume depletion.

Surgical procedures for lymphedema are classified as either excisional or physiologic. Excisional procedures remove diseased tissue; physiologic procedures attempt to restore lymph flow. Examples of excisional procedures include the Charles procedure in which all skin, subcutaneous tissue, and fascia are excised and a skin graft is applied to remaining muscle. Suction lipectomy works in some cases. Both require wearing a compression garment postoperatively. Physiologic procedures include microsurgical anastomosis of damaged lymphatic channels to veins, and fasciocutaneous or musculocutaneous flap transposition to an affected area to bring in new lymphatics. Overall, surgical therapies remain only marginally successful.

Thermal and Chemical Injuries

Jesse A. Taylor, MD

Thermal and chemical injuries are among the most severe traumatic events that a person can suffer and still survive. They cause severe local and systemic derangements in homeostasis. The management of a patient with thermal injury requires an understanding of the pathophysiology, diagnosis, and treatment not only of the local skin injury but also of the systemic hemodynamic, metabolic, nutritional, and psychological alterations.

THERMAL INJURIES

■ Epidemiology

There are 2 to 3 million thermal injuries in the United States each year. Five percent to ten percent of burn victims require hospital admission, and 5,000 to 6,000 die as a direct result of their thermal injury. These patients require 1 to 2 hospital days for each percentage of total body surface area (TBSA) burned. However, early treatment accounts for just one sixth of the total cost of care, which includes postdischarge rehabilitation and management of chronic disabilities.

Patient age, extent of burn, and burn depth are the primary determinants of acute mortality from thermal injury. With improvement in ICU care and the philosophy of early excision and grafting of wounds, the percentage of patients who die acutely from thermal injury has decreased significantly over the past 30 years; acute mortality is most frequently due to inhalation injury. Death during early recovery, largely due to sepsis, remains a challenge. Infection continues to be the leading cause of morbidity and mortality overall, with pulmonary infection the usual source.

No one is immune from thermal injury, but demographic data reveal four high-risk groups: the very young, the very old, the very unlucky, and the very careless. Children under 2 years of age and elderly persons are at particular risk for sustaining burns in domestic cooking and bathing accidents. Young adults are frequently burned on the job or while engaging in nefarious activities (i.e., playing with fire, illicit drugs). In fact, fully three fourths of adult burns are the result of the victim's own action. Extensive efforts have been made to diminish the incidence of thermal injuries through public education with varying results.

■ Pathophysiology

The extent of thermal injury is determined by the intensity of the source and the time of exposure. The affected area is divided into three concentric zones: coagulation, stasis, and hyperemia. The central **zone of coagulation** consists of nonviable tissue. It is surrounded by the **zone of stasis**, where delayed microcirculatory collapse secondary to endothelial damage often leads to ischemia and subsequent necrosis. The outermost **zone of hyperemia**, consists of vessels in a state of vasodilatation due to inflammatory mediators.

The systemic response to thermal injury is driven in part by the loss of the skin's function as the barrier to vapor loss and bacterial invasion. There are accelerated fluid losses, decreased host resistance to infection, release of inflammatory mediators from the injured tissue with microvascular and end-organ dysfunction, and bacterial overgrowth within the eschar (the dead tissue covering a burn), resulting in systemic infection. Edema in the tissue immediately surrounding the burn occurs secondary to local release of vasoactive mediators such as prostaglandins and oxygen radicals. When thermal injury extends over 20% of total body surface area (TBSA), inflammatory mediators are released in sufficient quantities to cause a more global systemic inflammatory response syndrome (SIRS). Distant microvascular injury may interfere with the function of organ systems not directly related to the site of thermal injury, accounting for the frequent occurrence of pulmonary and other end-organ dysfunction with large burns. Other metabolic responses not entirely understood, but clinically significant, are endocrinopathy (altered hypothalamic-adrenal axis, insulin resistance), generalized edema, and deficient gastrointestinal barrier function with translocation of bacteria.

■ Diagnosis

Changing perfusion and thus viability in the zone of stasis and nonuniformity of burn depth make it difficult to accurately determine extent and depth of burn within the first 24 hours. Many techniques to assist in diagnosis of depth of injury have been developed, including burn biopsy, laser Doppler flowmeter, and fluorescein dye, but none has been as accurate as clinical observation by an experienced burn specialist. Table 5-1 reviews the classical anatomy and characteristics of differing burn depths.

■ TABLE 5-1 Classification of Burn Depth

Burn Degree	Anatomic Depth	Surface Appearance	Pain Level
First degree (superficial)	Through epidermis	Dry; no blisters; reddish (e.g., sunburn)	Painful
Second degree (partial thickness)	Involving dermis	Moist blebs; blisters; mottled white to pink	Very painful
Third degree (full thickness)	Through dermis and into subcutaneous	Dry with leathery eschar; waxy, white, dark khaki	No pain; hair pulls out easily
Fourth degree (full thickness)	Involves underlying structures such as muscle and bone	Same as third degree; exposed bone, muscle, or tendon	Same as third degree

Functionally, it is helpful to think of burns as being epidermal, dermal (superficial or deep), or full-thickness because of differences in method of healing.

Extent of burn in adults is estimated by the "rule of 9's." In humans it is estimated that a person's palm of the hand is equivalent to 1% TBSA. The surface area of the other major parts of the body is divided into multiples of 9. The head represents 9% of the body surface, and each arm is 9%. The front of each leg is 9%, and the back 9%. The front of the torso is 18%, and the back is 18%. Burn centers use standardized graphics to illustrate the extent of burn.

■ Treatment

Victims of thermal injury often sustain additional injuries, and should be evaluated like any victim of multiple trauma. Advanced trauma life support (ATLS) guidelines begin with a primary survey, effective airway and vascular access, and a systemic secondary survey. Severe burns demand "a tube in every orifice," including endotracheal tube, nasogastric tube, Foley catheter, and at least two large-bore IV lines. Tetanus prophylaxis is standard of care. The American Burn Association (ABA) has developed criteria for referral to a specialized burn center (Box 5-1).

Initial Management of Victims of Thermal Injury

■ History

Ascertain closed space exposure, time of exposure, prehospital management, past medical history, medications, and allergies.

■ BOX 5-1 Patients Requiring Burn Unit Care (ABA Criteria)

1. Partial-thickness and full-thickness burns >10% TBSA in patients <10 or >50 years of age
2. Partial-thickness and full-thickness burns >20% TBSA in any age group
3. Burns that involve the face, hands, feet, genitalia, perineum, or major joints
4. Full-thickness burns >5% in any age group
5. Any electrical or chemical burn
6. Burn injury in patients with complicating, preexisting medical disorders
7. Any patients with burns and concomitant trauma in which the burn injury poses the greatest risk for morbidity and mortality

■ Pulmonary

Assess airway control, chest excursion, and the need for thoracic escharotomy.

Inhalational Injury

This is a major source of mortality from thermal injury.

- **Pathogenesis**: (1) direct thermal injury to the upper aerodigestive tract, (2) inhalation of products of combustion that chemically burn the lower tracheobronchial tree, (3) carbon monoxide inhalation.
- **Diagnosis**: physical examination; singed nasal hairs, facial or oropharyngeal burns, carbonaceous sputum, stridor; arterial blood gas (ABG) analysis, including carboxyhemoglobin levels (CHgb > 10% significant; CHgb > 50% associated with high mortality); serial ABGs necessary because oxygen saturation can be artificially elevated in the setting of high concentrations of CHgb.
- **Treatment**: supportive; endotracheal intubation; administration of 100% oxygen (which decreases the washout time of CO from 250 minutes to 40–50 minutes); frequent nasotracheal suctioning of carbonaceous materials to prevent mucous plugging; aggressive treatment of infectious pulmonary complications.

■ Cardiovascular/Fluid Resuscitation

Massive fluid, electrolyte, and protein losses can be expected in the acute setting. High volume fluid resuscitation is needed to avoid "burn shock." Reliable signs of adequate perfusion are neurologic function (arousable, oriented), urine output (adults 0.5 mL/kg/hr, children 1 mL/kg/hr), and vital signs (heart rate, blood pressure). Patients with renal failure or heart failure may require advanced monitoring by central venous catheter or Swan-Ganz catheter. The Parkland formula (Table 5-2) has been developed as

■ **TABLE 5-2 Parkland Formula**	
Day 1	Lactated Ringer's solution: Total volume = 4 mL/kg/% TBSA burn Give $1/2$ in first 8 h; give $1/2$ over the next 16 h
Day 2	Switch to D5W and adjust based on urine output Begin albumin* 5% in mL/h = (0.5–1.0 mL/kg/%TBSA burn)/16
Day 3	Change to maintenance IV fluid and adjust based on urine output[†] Attempt to start enteral nutrition

*The administration of albumin in burn patients is controversial and is therefore done on a selective basis in many burn centers.
[†]Urine output is the primary determinant of hydration status and trumps the Parkland formula.

a guideline to estimate fluid requirements in the severely burned patient.

■ Upper Airway

Perioral and intraoral burns, carbonaceous sputum, and progressive hoarseness indicate airway involvement. Early management is focused on securing the airway with endotracheal intubation as needed.

■ Laboratory Examination

Arterial blood gas (with carboxyhemoglobin level) is important when airway compromise or inhalation injury is present. Baseline hemoglobin and electrolytes may be helpful during resuscitation. Urinalysis for occult blood should be performed with deep thermal or electrical injuries.

■ Abdomen

A nasogastric tube should be placed and its function verified. Immediate stress ulcer prophylaxis with histamine receptor blockers is indicated with serious burns. Abdominal escharotomy may facilitate ventilation.

■ Extremities

Extremities with circumferential burns should be promptly decompressed by escharotomy when clinical examination reveals diminished distal perfusion. Medial and lateral axial approaches to escharotomy are recommended. Fasciotomy is rarely necessary except in fourth-degree burns and electrical injuries. Limbs at risk should be dressed so they can be frequently examined. Burned extremities should be elevated and splinted in a position of function.

■ **Wounds**

Size, depth, and presence of circumferential burns should be determined immediately and with caution. Wounds are often underestimated in depth and overestimated in size on initial examination. Adequate analgesia must be given before initial débridement of loose skin and gentle washing of the wounds. After necrotic tissue has been removed, a topical agent is applied (Table 5-3). Topical antimicrobials have revolutionized the treatment of burns, greatly diminishing the prevalence of burn wound sepsis. *Note: There is no role for prophylactic use of systemic antibiotics to prevent burn wound sepsis.*

■ **Nutrition**

The hypermetabolic response to burn injury is intense and requires full support from the day of injury throughout the period of wound closure. Metabolic rate is proportional to TBSA burned, and may be as much as twice the basal energy expenditure (BEE). Useful guidelines for predicting the nutritional needs of severely burned patients include the Harris-Benedict equation and the Curreri formula. Of the routes of providing nutrients, enteral feeding is preferred for its lower infection rates, decreased cost, and decreased complications.

■ TABLE 5-3 Topical Antimicrobial Agents in Burn Care	
Silver sulfadiazine (Silvadene)	Painless on application, nonstaining, applied b.i.d. No metabolic side effects Broad antimicrobial spectrum, rare resistance Moderate eschar penetration Can form pseudoeschar that can limit penetration Common side effect: self-limited leukopenia, sulfa hypersensitivity reaction
Silver nitrate	Painless on application, stains brown Leeches electrolytes Broad antimicrobial spectrum, rare resistance Poor eschar penetration Dressings must be kept wet—time intensive Major side effect: methemoglobinemia; electrolyte depletion
Mafenide acetate (Sulfamylon)	Painful on application, applied b.i.d. Excellent eschar and cartilage penetration (ears, nose) Broad antimicrobial spectrum Common side effect: diuresis and acid/base abnormalities may be caused by this carbonic anhydrase inhibitor

Burn Wound Care

The goal of burn wound care is early excision of necrotic tissue and coverage of burn wounds to minimize infection, pain, and morbidity. First-degree burns require pain control and minimal local wound care. Superficial second-degree burns require an initial washing with antiseptic soap, removal of debris, unroofing of vesicles, and application of topical agents (Table 5-3). Deep second-degree burns and full-thickness burns require local wound care followed by excision and grafting.

Historically, major burns were treated for a period of 2 to 3 weeks with local wound care prior to excision and grafting. In 1970 the philosophy of excision and grafting within the first 2 to 7 days revolutionized the care of burn patients. Although this change in management has decreased overall mortality only slightly, it has resulted in a major reduction in morbidity as defined by cost of care, length of hospitalization, loss of job productivity, pain, and chronic disability. Physiologically, it reduces overall necrotic tissue load and the incidence of burn wound sepsis. Early wound stabilization facilitates early joint mobility with less stiffness and ultimately improved function. Finally, it restores the primary barrier to dehydration and infection.

■ Order of Excision in Major Burn Injuries

The order of excision in major burns requires the judgment of an experienced burn surgeon. The clinical condition and premorbid function of the patient must be taken into account. There are two competing schools of thought regarding order of excision:

1. Highest priority is to **diminish overall necrotic tissue load and minimize infection**. Broad areas like the trunk and extremities are given priority for excision.
2. Highest priority is to graft areas that will give the patient the **highest functionality** and **best cosmetic outcome**. Thus, hand, feet, joints, extremities, and face are grafted first.

■ Technique of Excision

There are two techniques of excision of burn eschar: tangential excision and fascial excision. Tangential excision is performed the majority of the time, while fascial excision is reserved for limited indications.

Tangential excision is the removal of thin layers of necrotic tissue, one layer at a time, until punctate, uniform, brisk bleeding is seen. Manual dermatomes (Humby, Goulian) are preferred for small, irregular surfaces like the hands and face. Electric or compressed air dermatomes are preferred for uniform, large surfaces like the trunk and legs. Bleeding may be controlled by excising under tourniquet control or by covering excised areas with a laparotomy pad soaked in 1:200,000 epinephrine solution.

Fascial excision is reserved for very deep burns and large, life-threatening, full-thickness burns. Excision is carried out with a scalpel or electrocautery to the level of the fascia. Although this type of excision is fast and produces a reliable tissue bed for grafting, it also results in poor appearance and risks damage to superficial structures such as nerves, vessels, and subcutaneous padding of joints.

■ Choice of Graft

The goal of burn surgery is to excise and autograft (patient's own skin) all deep dermal and deeper burns. In the absence of sufficient skin for autografting, the best option for wound coverage after massive burn excision is **cadaver allograft** (banked human skin). Table 5-4 reviews other physiologic dressings that can temporarily cover the wound until definitive closure, that is, until autografting is possible.

■ Autograft Variables

Thickness of Graft (Split Thickness versus Full Thickness)
The numerous issues surrounding choice of graft thickness are discussed in Chapter 3 and include rates of primary and secondary contraction, donor site morbidity, graft survival rates, pigmentation, and sensation. Split-thickness skin grafts are used almost exclusively in acute burn management.

■ TABLE 5-4 Temporary Wound Dressings			
Material	**Source**	**Advantages**	**Disadvantages**
Allograft	Banked human skin	Angiogenic; incorporates into wound; means of testing whether a marginal bed will take an autograft	Expensive; must be kept frozen and thawed in advance; comes in small sizes; is rejected at 1 wk
Biobrane	Nylon and silicon	Elastic, uniform, transparent, readily available	Difficult to use, does not incorporate into wound and is variably adherent; infection
Xenograft	Pig skin	Effective; readily available; comes in large sizes	Biodegradable; does not incorporate into wound

Sheet Graft versus Mesh Graft

Because a wound is reepithelialized from the edges, the perimeter of the graft is the only part that contributes to the epithelialization process. This principle has led burn surgeons to mesh, or cut slits in, skin grafts to increase the surface area that participates in reepithelialization. Meshed grafts are larger and more pliable than their nonmeshed counterparts. They have a lower incidence of seroma or hematoma formation because their interstices provide drainage. That said, most sheet grafts are perforated in some fashion to allow for efflux of effluent. Bacterial contamination is isolated by the mesh effect, so there is less chance of losing the entire graft due to infection. The disadvantages of meshing are the considerable surface area that must heal by secondary intention and the poor, "pebbled" appearance of a meshed graft. These disadvantages are minimized by using a small ratio of expansion (for instance 1:1.5) and by pulling the graft lengthwise to narrow the skin perforations.

Skin Graft Fixation

Multiple options exist for securing the graft, and the choice is usually based on location and size of the graft, as well as surgeon preference. Examples include suture materials (Chromic, nylon), tissue adhesives, skin staples, and Steri-Strips.

Complications (Ch. 3)

Common causes of graft failure are seroma, hematoma, mechanical sheer, and infection. Inadequacy of the graft bed either due to lack of adequate blood supply or presence of necrotic tissue also can contribute to graft failure.

■ Cultured Epithelial Autografts

Cultured epithelial autografts (CEAs) are useful in the setting of massive burn with limited donor site availability. Functional "grafts" are grown in culture from individual epithelial cells taken from a biopsy of a patient's skin or oral mucosa. In 2 weeks' time they grow to cover an area as much as 10,000 times the original area of the biopsy. Once the CEA cells take, they will spread peripherally to join other grafts or surrounding skin. CEAs are extremely fragile and quite expensive, with a 4 × 4 cm graft costing over $600. CEAs are also very sensitive to infection, tolerating maximum bacterial counts of 10^2 to $10^3/cm^3$ (compared with $10^5/cm^3$ for standard split-thickness skin grafts).

■ Donor Site Management

The goal of donor site management is to obtain a **fast rate of healing** that is **painless**, **cost effective**, and **free from infection**. Synthetic wound dressings available for donor site coverage are classified as semiopen, semiocclusive, and occlusive. Semiopen dressings like impregnated gauze (Scarlet Red, Vaseline gauze) and biobrane are relatively cheap, provide healing in 1 to 2 weeks, but cause moderate pain. Generally, they are dried with a hair dryer to produce an artificial "scab" that falls off as the wound heals. Alternatively, semiocclusive dressings like OpSite and Tegaderm provide more rapid rates of healing and minimal pain at a moderate price. Their drawback is that they can be difficult to apply and are susceptible to bacterial contamination through leaks. If malpositioned, they must be considered contaminated and replaced with a semiopen dressing. Occlusive dressings like Duoderm are rarely used because they are expensive and difficult to use.

A rare but devastating complication is donor site infection that transforms a partial-thickness donor site into a full-thickness wound. Treatment consists of antibiotics, débridement of necrotic tissue, and excision and grafting.

■ Graft Site Management

Postoperative management of skin grafts is an area where there are many opinions and few data. Some centers use wet, antibiotic-soaked gauze over nonstick Adaptic gauze and frequently wrap these with ACE bandages for light compression. The operative dressing is left in place for 3 days then changed daily thereafter. Daily changes provide gentle crust débridement. It is common to use wet dressings until the interstices of the grafts have reepithelialized. As the graft matures and is more durable, there is a transition from Xeroform gauze or Bacitracin to no coverage. Sheet grafts are left open to air for frequent inspection.

■ Management of Specific Areas

Ears

The most important factor in treating ear burns is prevention of suppurative chondritis, which is exceedingly painful, requires débridement of all involved cartilage, and can be quite deforming. Prevention involves avoiding pressure on the ear and topical antimicrobial therapy with **Mafenide** because of its excellent cartilage penetration. Suppurative chondritis mandates immediate débridement of cartilage and systemic antibiotic therapy (*Pseudomonas* is the usual infecting organism).

Eyelids

Eyelid burns frequently result in ectropion and exposure of the globe. Proper treatment includes lubrication followed by thick split-thickness skin graft or full-thickness skin graft from the contralateral eyelid, postauricular area, or groin. Tarsorrhaphy is rarely helpful, and more often results in injury to the tarsal plate as contraction forces pull out tarsorrhaphy sutures.

Face
Full-thickness burns to the face are tangentially excised and sheet grafted in aesthetic units. Often a two-staged procedure is performed with excision and allografting followed by autografting 24 to 72 hours later. This is a formidable undertaking in terms of blood loss and postoperative care. Postoperatively the patient is sedated for 5 days, during which he or she is tube fed, and not allowed to chew or talk (some surgeons even apply intermaxillary fixation). Grafts are inspected frequently, and fluid collections aspirated. One week postoperatively, the patient is custom fitted with a Uvex face mask to wear while the grafts mature. In the long term, skin grafts are aesthetically suboptimal, and many patients choose to undergo delayed flap reconstruction to improve their appearance.

Hands
Indeterminate or full-thickness hand burns are aggressively excised and grafted early to preserve maximal function and cause the shortest disability from these wounds. Although palmar burns rarely need grafting because of the protective fist-clenching reaction to injury, dorsal burns are sheet grafted to minimize healing time and contraction. Dressings are applied over the grafts incorporating a previously fabricated Orthoplast splint. Exposed bones, tendons, and joints require flap coverage.

Lower Extremity
Burns to the lower extremities below the knee are particularly difficult to heal because of dependent edema and increased infection rates. Because of their problematic nature, some burn centers admit to the hospital all burns below the knees.

ELECTRICAL INJURIES

■ Epidemiology
Acute electrical injuries account for approximately 2% of burn center admissions. About 15% have suffered additional multisystem trauma, and require ATLS resuscitation. Although the mean TBSA burn is only about 10% to 15%, the cutaneous injury usually does not reflect the extent of deep tissue damage.

■ Pathophysiology
Tissue damage in electrical injury occurs as electrical current is transformed into heat. The most severely affected areas are the entry and exit sites, where electrical current is most concentrated.

The effects of passage of current through the body depend on the **type of circuit** (destruction of tissue greater with alternating current than direct current), **the voltage of the circuit**, **duration of contact**, **pathway of current through the body**, and **resistance offered by tissues**. With greater resistance, more heat is generated. There is a ranking of body tissue resistance from greatest to least: bone > fat > tendon > skin > muscle > vessel. As with burns, microvascular injury and thrombosis magnifies tissue destruction.

■ Diagnosis

Multiple types of injury may result from exposure to high-voltage electricity. The entry and exit points typically manifest local cutaneous injury, whereas current passing through deep tissues causes deeper injury. Flame burns occur when clothing ignites. Intense contraction of paravertebral muscles may cause spine fractures. Fall- and blast-related injuries also frequently accompany high-voltage injury.

Commonly, there is progressive loss of viable tissue in the first few days following an electrical injury. Muscle, especially, may appear viable on immediate exploration and nonviable on delayed exploration. Exact delineation of damaged muscle can be ascertained with a technetium-99m stannous pyrophosphate muscle scan.

■ Treatment

All electrical injuries require full ATLS resuscitation, including cardiac monitoring, bladder catheterization to evaluate the urine for pigment, and spine immobilization pending radiographic examination of the axial spine. Edematous injured muscle can cause elevated compartment pressure and additional ischemia. At risk areas must be carefully monitored for pressure elevation and need for release.

Fluid replacement is calculated from the size of the cutaneous injury plus an additional amount based on hypothesized deep tissue injury. In the presence of gross urinary pigment, 2 ampoules of sodium bicarbonate and 2 ampoules of mannitol are added to each liter of IV fluids in order to increase urine output and alkalinize the urine to prevent myoglobin crystal precipitation (rhabdomyolysis) and renal failure. Resuscitation goals include a urine output of 100 mL/hr in the adult and 1.5 to 2 mL/kg/hr in children.

Operative débridement is the definitive therapy for electric injuries. Because of the threat of delayed injury, often multiple operative sessions are required to adequately débride all necrotic tissue and avoid sepsis. The application of topical agents with excellent eschar penetration, like Mafenide, supplements surgical therapy.

CHEMICAL INJURIES

Chemical burns involve alkalis, acids, or organic compounds. Alkaline substances such as sodium and potassium hydroxides and cements are the most common causes. The severity of chemical injury is related to the nature of the agent, its concentration, and the volume and duration of contact. The outcome of an injury is directly proportional to the amount of time of chemical contact.

■ Treatment

Patients who suffer chemical burns are initially treated with **copious tap water irrigation** to dilute and neutralize the offending agent. Ocular injuries are irrigated with saline. Topical ophthalmic anesthetics facilitate relief of the blepharospasm that often interferes with effective irrigation of the globe. Several chemical burns require specific antidotes.

- **Hydrofluoric acid**—Patients may experience life-threatening hypocalcemia. Burns are treated with 10% calcium gluconate paste applied to the affected area; severe cases require subeschar injection of calcium gluconate.
- **Phenol**—Phenol is not soluble in water and requires topical application of polyethylene glycol or vegetable oil for neutralization.
- **Phosphorous**—Phosphorous burns must be kept continuously wet with water to prevent particle desiccation and ignition. Copper sulfate (2%) aids in diagnosis by turning phosphorous particles black in color. Early surgical débridement of extraneous particles is the cornerstone of therapy.
- **Cement**—Cement burns are irrigated copiously with water until the soapy feeling has disappeared and then the area is dried thoroughly.
- **Tar**—Tar burns are initially cooled by tap water irrigation to limit the progression of the injury. The tar is later removed by lipophilic solvent. They respond well to application of Bacitracin ointment and Silvadene.

REHABILITATION

As postburn survival becomes the rule rather than the exception, more emphasis is being placed on quality of life issues. Dedicated burn occupational and physical therapists facilitate return to optimal function by remaining involved through the acute injury resuscitation and continuing after discharge.

Psychosocial adaptation after severe burns remains a challenge, especially if the hands and face are involved. The coordinated involvement of psychiatric, psychological, and social work staff facilitates maximal recovery and social reintegration. These staff should be actively involved with the patient, family, and local outpatient support services throughout the hospitalization. The expectation for every burn patient should be a return to family and mainstream community life.

RECONSTRUCTION

As in other areas of plastic surgery, the goal of postburn reconstruction is to restore form and function of affected areas. Wound contracture and hypertrophic scar formation are two processes that plague burn patients long term.

Myofibroblasts are responsible for contracture that may limit mobility. This may be intrinsic or extrinsic distortion of tissues. Intrinsic contracture results from direct contracture of a region and requires reconstruction with a graft or flap. Extrinsic contracture results from contracture of an adjacent body part and requires release—for example, ectropion from a burn of the cheek.

Hypertrophic scars are both cosmetically unappealing and functionally limiting. They occur most frequently in young, dark-skinned patients with deep dermal burns that were grafted more than 3 weeks after injury. Grafting earlier minimizes hypertrophy. Wounds in areas of tension such as the flexor surfaces, the anterior neck, and the submental area are also at a greater risk for hypertrophy. Current prophylaxis includes compression garments, silicone gel sheeting, and steroid injections. Compression garments are custom fitted and are worn from the time the graft is deemed stable until it is fully mature. The mechanism of action of silicone gel sheeting is unclear and is accompanied by frequent skin irritation and rashes. Judicious intradermal steroid injection is useful in the management of limited areas of hypertrophic scarring, usually in small, cosmetically sensitive areas. Patients with recalcitrant areas of hypertrophic scarring are best served by release or excision and grafting. Resultant wounds are covered with sheet autograft or flaps. Tissue expanders (Chapter 3) can be of great value, particularly in the closure of defects adjacent to large areas of normal soft tissue.

When function is not threatened, it is best to wait until a scar is fully mature before embarking on reconstructive procedures. In most cases this means waiting at least a year. Prompt surgery is indicated when function is threatened. Patients with large burn wounds commonly require a series of reconstructive procedures during the first few years after injury to attain the best possible cosmetic and functional results.

6 Craniofacial Surgery

Thomas X. Hahm, MD and Jesse A. Taylor, MD

Embryology and Anatomy

In the third week of development, an embryo's primitive ecto-dermal layer splits to form cutaneous and neural structures. The neural tube is formed at this stage, the boundary of which is termed the neural crest. Neural crest cells migrate to various loca-tions in the head and neck and differentiate into specialized structures. Failure of this migration or differentiation is the pathologic basis for most craniofacial deformities.

The face is formed from five facial prominences: the fron-tonasal prominence, paired maxillary prominences, and paired mandibular prominences. The frontonasal prominence becomes the forehead, nasal dorsum, and medial and lateral nasal promi-nences. The maxillary prominences form most of the upper mid-face and upper lip. A cleft lip results when the medial nasal prominence fails to fuse with the maxillary prominence. The mandibular prominences form much of the lower third of the face. The maxillary and mandibular prominences fuse laterally to form the oral commissure.

The neonatal calvarium is composed of the following bone plates: frontal, parietal, temporal, sphenoid and occipital. There are seven suture lines located at the junction of the bone plates, which are the growth centers of the developing cranium. The metopic suture separates the frontal bones and is the first to fuse, or disappear, at 2 years of age. The coronal suture separates the frontal bone from the parietal bones. The sagittal suture separates the two parietal bones. The squamosal suture lies between the parietal and temporal bones. Finally the lambdoid suture lies between the parietal and occipital bones.

Craniosynostosis

Craniosynostosis is the pathologic premature fusion of cranial sutures, resulting in restriction of growth perpendicular to the involved suture and compensatory growth parallel to it. This results in an abnormally shaped skull.

■ Etiology

The complex biology of suture growth and closure is under investigation; currently the cause of premature closure of one or more cranial sutures is unknown. Interactions between cranial sutures and the meninges may play an important role in sutural closure. Some believe that genetics plays a role, as well.

■ Diagnosis

The diagnosis of craniosynostosis is usually made by a parent or primary care physician at birth or early in infancy. A detailed history and physical is followed by genetic counseling, a search for intracranial abnormalities, and the development of a treatment plan. CT scans of the head and face guide diagnosis and treatment. Three-dimensional CT scans are helpful in reconstructive planning. Table 6-1 reviews the various types of craniosynostosis.

■ Treatment

Methods of treatment range from positional therapy, to molding helmets, to surgery. Surgical intervention is indicated to relieve increased intracranial pressure or to produce an aesthetically acceptable cranial vault. Surgical treatment consists of a series of osteotomies and bone reshaping followed by rigid fixation of bone.

Craniosynostosis Syndromes

■ Apert's Syndrome

Apert's syndrome is characterized by craniosynostosis, exorbitism, midface hypoplasia, and symmetric syndactyly (digital fusion) of hands and feet. Acne vulgaris is a distinguishing feature in the condition. Although mental retardation is common among Apert's patients, some have normal mental function. Most cases are sporadic, but autosomal-dominant transmission has been described.

■ Crouzon's Syndrome

Similar to Apert's syndrome, Crouzon's syndrome is characterized by craniosynostosis, midface hypoplasia, and ocular proptosis. The absence of syndactyly or other limb anomalies and the predominance of normal mental function distinguishes Crouzon's from Apert's. The mode of transmission is autosomal dominant.

■ Pfeiffer's Syndrome

Pfeiffer's syndrome consists of craniosynostosis and broad-based toes and thumbs. Maxillary hypoplasia with shallow orbits and proptosis is also common. The affected subjects usually have normal intellect. The mode of transmission is autosomal dominant.

■ TABLE 6-1 Craniosynostoses

Suture Prematurely Fused	Name of Craniosynostosis	Features	Goals of Treatment
Metopic (10% of cases)	Trigonocephaly (keel-shaped skull)	Midline forehead ridge, bitemporal narrowing and hypertelorism	Correct orbital rim abnormality, expand the anterior cranial vault
Sagittal (most common)	Scaphocephaly (Greek *scapha* = boat)	Decreased skull width and increased length	Increase temporal and parietal width, reduce skull length
Unilateral coronal	Plagiocephaly (Greek *plagio* = oblique)	Flattened forehead, harlequin eye deformity, elevation of ipsilateral ear	Expand anterior cranial vault, advance ipsilateral orbit, establish symmetric forehead
Bilateral coronal	Brachycephaly (Greek *brachy* = short)	Shortened anteroposterior length, transverse widening, vertical elongation, orbital rim hypoplasia, occipital flattening	Decrease skull height, increase anterior cranial vault, advance orbital rims
Lambdoid (rare)	Posterior plagiocephaly	Flattening of affected occiput, distortion of cranial base, posteroinferior displacement of ear	Expand posterior cranial vault*

*True lambdoid synostosis must be distinguished from positional posterior plagiocephaly, a benign condition caused by constant pressure on the occiput (baby sleeping supine constantly). Positional posterior plagiocephaly is treated by changing the baby's sleeping position—surgery is not indicated.

Sathre-Chotzen Syndrome

The syndrome consists of craniosynostosis, low-set hairline, and ptosis of the eyelids. The mode of transmission is autosomal dominant with variable penetrance. The low-set hairline is the pathognomic feature.

Carpenter's Syndrome

Carpenter's syndrome is characterized by craniosynostosis, brachydactyly (short fingers), syndactyly (fused fingers usually only soft tissue), polydactyly (numerous digits), and low-set ears. Congenital heart anomalies have also been described. The mode of transmission is sporadic in most cases, but autosomal-recessive inheritance has been described. The defining feature is low-set ears.

Treacher-Collins Syndrome

Treacher-Collins syndrome, also known as mandibulofacial dysostosis, is representative of Tessier's clefts 6, 7, and 8. Its pattern of inheritance is autosomal dominant with an incidence of 1 in 10,000 live births. The clinical features are mental retardation, downward-slanting eyes, colobomas of the lower lid, malar hypoplasia, mandibular hypoplasia, macrostomia, high arched palate, ear malformations, and absence of eyelashes in the medial third of the lower eyelid.

Nager's Anomaly

A much rarer relative of Treacher-Collins syndrome, Nager's anomaly has an autosomal-recessive inheritance. Additional features are hypoplasia or agenesis of the thumbs, radius, and metacarpals.

Cleft Lip and Palate

Epidemiology

Cleft lip with or without cleft palate occurs in 1 in 700 live births. Cleft lip is most common in Asians followed by whites then blacks. The incidence of isolated cleft palate is 1 in 2,500 live births and is constant across races. If one child is affected, the risk of a second child developing cleft lip or palate is around 4%. If a parent and a child are affected, the risk for a future child developing cleft lip or palate is around 15%. Approximately 10% of patients born with cleft lip or palate have associated anomalies.

Etiology

The etiology of cleft lip and palate is multifactorial, with varying contributions from genetics and the environment. Studies of multiple environmental factors such as maternal smoking, alcoholism, and caffeine abuse have not clearly determined an association. However, nutritional deficiencies of vitamins like folate have been associated with higher rates of cleft lip and palate. Corticosteroid use during pregnancy has also been associated.

■ Diagnosis

Embryologically, cleft lip develops at 4 to 6 weeks, whereas cleft palate develops later, at 7 to 12 weeks. Thus, cleft lip and palate can be diagnosed by transvaginal ultrasonography as early as the first trimester of pregnancy. That said, the majority of cases are diagnosed by physical examination at birth.

Multiple classification schemes exist, and most are quite complex. Simply put, cleft lip can be classified as unilateral or bilateral, and complete or incomplete. Similarly, cleft palate can be classified as unilateral or bilateral, complete or incomplete, and isolated or in conjunction with cleft lip (Figures 6-1 and 6-2).

■ Treatment

The treatment of cleft lip and palate requires a dedicated, multidisciplinary team composed of speech therapists, orthodontists, and surgeons. Cleft lips are repaired in the first 6 months of life for both aesthetic and physiologic reasons. Repair usually requires the rotation and advancement of surrounding structures to achieve coaptation of oral mucosa, orbicularis oris muscle, and skin of appropriate dimensions.

Cleft palates are repaired around the first birthday to allow for normal development of speech and feeding patterns. Again, repair usually involves the rotation or advancement of surrounding structures to achieve palatal closure. Secondary bone grafting of the hard palate is done during the period of mixed dentition, or around ages 4 to 7. About 80% of cleft palate repairs result in palatal competency; the remaining 20% of cases require a secondary

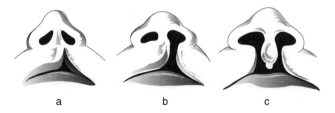

a   b   c

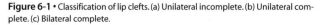

Figure 6-1 • Classification of lip clefts. (a) Unilateral incomplete. (b) Unilateral complete. (c) Bilateral complete.

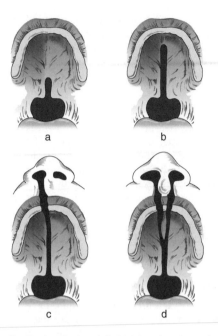

Figure 6-2 • Classification of palate clefts. (a) Palate alone, incomplete. (b) Palate alone, complete. (c) Unilateral complete cleft lip and palate. (d) Bilateral complete cleft lip and palate.

procedure to treat velopharyngeal incompetence (inability for the palate and pharynx to form a sealed valve).

Craniofacial Clefts

As stated previously, craniofacial clefts represent a failure of the facial prominences to fuse as well as failure of differentiation of neural crest cells. Craniofacial clefts are exceedingly rare and are usually treated by specialized teams of physicians at tertiary care centers.

Nomenclature is based on Tessier's classification system for facial clefts which assigns clefts a number from 0 to 14 based on their position relative to the midline. Clefts of the upper face are numbered 9 to 14; those of the lower face are numbered 0 to 8. Clefts may be isolated, appear in tandem, or appear as part of a craniofacial syndrome. Thus, the presence of a facial cleft should prompt genetic analysis as well as thorough workup of the craniofacial skeleton and soft tissues.

Hemifacial Microsomia

■ Epidemiology

The incidence of hemifacial microsomia is 1 in 4,000 live births, with 10% occurring bilaterally. There is no evidence of genetic transmission, and males seem to be affected more than females.

■ Etiology

The exact etiology is not known, but the most widely held hypothesis is that of a vascular insult to the first and second branchial arches early in their development with subsequent hypoplasia of affected structures. Depending on the timing and location of the hypothesized vascular accident, the syndrome may take on a spectrum of severity.

■ Clinical Presentation

The expression of the syndrome is variable, and thus can range from mild forms such as preauricular skin tags or microtia, to full expression of complete soft tissue and skeletal deficits. Severe cases exhibit mandibular hypoplasia with chin deviation toward the affected side, midface hypoplasia, microtia, facial nerve palsy, and severe soft tissue deficits.

■ Treatment

Treatment depends on the clinical expression. Airway management is a top priority and usually involves displacing the tongue and enlarging the mandible. Grafts and free tissue transfers are frequently used when severe bony and soft tissue deficits are encountered. Distraction osteogenesis has become a popular method of treating the micrognathia associated with hemifacial microsomia. Prosthetics are helpful adjuncts to surgery.

Goldenhar's Syndrome

Goldenhar's syndrome is a sporadic anomaly closely resembling hemifacial microsomia. Additional features include vertebral anomalies, epibulbar dermoids, and colobomas of the upper eyelid.

Encephaloceles

An encephalocele is a congenital malformation characterized by a protrusion of cranial contents through a skull defect. Encephaloceles are due to a failure of regression of a dural projection through the skull, the reasons for which are unknown. They are classified based on their location and contents. The skull defect occurs in two main places: the frontoethmoidal region and the occipital region. It may contain meninges (meningocele), brain (encephalomeningocele), or ventricle (encephalomeningocystocele).

Treatment consists of resection of excess dura mater, reduction of herniated intracranial components, and watertight closure of the dura. Soft tissue and bony reconstruction are performed as needed.

Romberg's Disease

Progressive hemifacial atrophy, or **Romberg's disease**, is a rare hemifacial atrophic condition that typically begins in the first or second decade of life. The etiology is unknown, and it can present bilaterally. The process starts in the subcutaneous tissue then progresses to the muscle, the bones, and even the skin. Treatment is directed at restoring the volume discrepancy or deficiency. Reconstructive methods include fat injections, facial prosthetic implants, and local flaps. Microsurgical free tissue transfers are performed for severe cases.

Fibrous Dysplasia

Fibrous dysplasia is a condition involving an abnormal increase in bone forming mesenchyme leading to bony overgrowth. Histologically, there is an arrest of bone maturation leading to immature bony deposition. Malignant degeneration occurs in less than 0.5% of cases. Two forms of fibrous dysplasia exist, monostotic (single bone) and polyostotic (multiple bones). The ribs and femur are the most common sites affected, followed by skull, maxilla, and mandible.

Treatment involves surgical resection, although there is a high recurrence rate. No medical treatment at this time has been effective, and radiation therapy is contraindicated because it can incite malignant degeneration.

Facial Trauma

■ Early Management

Facial trauma commonly occurs in the setting of multisystem trauma, and patients must be treated according to ATLS guidelines. Blood, vomitus, and soft tissue which compromise the airway are cleared. There is a low threshold for intubation.

Once the airway is secured, the circulatory system is evaluated. Facial injuries are commonly associated with massive bleeding.

Superficial bleeding is usually controlled with manual pressure. Bleeding from the nose may require a combination of anterior and posterior nasal packing. Uncontrolled bleeding from deep structures requires either angiographic embolization or operative intervention.

■ Diagnosis and Treatment

A thorough survey of the head and neck is made before proceeding with definitive treatment. All lacerations, abrasions, and puncture wounds are critically examined for injury to adjacent nerves (cranial nerves II–VII), arteries, or other structures (lacrimal apparatus around the eye, parotid duct in the cheek). Soft tissue injuries are irrigated copiously, débrided minimally, and closed primarily. Suggestions for closure of specific areas are found in Chapter 1.

Underlying fractures are identified by physical examination and appropriate radiographic examination, usually a CT scan. Cervical spine and intracranial pathology frequently accompany facial fractures, and thorough examination is required prior to initiating definitive treatment. Ophthalmologists, dentists, and neurosurgeons are consulted as needed.

Facial fractures are classified anatomically as closed or open, displaced or nondisplaced, simple or comminuted, and functionally impairing or not. Absolute indications for facial fracture repair are uncontrolled hemorrhage caused by a fracture, acute airway compromise, and entrapment of orbital soft tissues within a fracture leading to diplopia with upward gaze. Relative indications for facial fracture repair include functional and aesthetic deformities described below.

Facial bones are arranged such that thickened areas of strong bone are aligned to create vertical and horizontal buttresses. Bony fixation is concentrated on these areas of strength, because these areas primarily give the face its shape. Common strategies for facial fracture repair include splinting, closed reduction, and open reduction with internal fixation. Best results have been achieved when early operative intervention is used.

Frontal Sinus Fractures

The paired frontal sinuses develop around 5 to 10 years of age to occupy the lower third of the frontal bone. They have an anterior and posterior table, a midline bony septum, and a thickened inferior aspect that forms the superior orbital rims. Fluid produced by their mucosa drains through the floor of the sinuses into the middle meatus of the nose via the nasofrontal ducts. Fractures of the frontal sinuses are usually asymptomatic and must be suspected in patients with forehead lacerations or bruising. A facial CT scan usually confirms the diagnosis.

Closed, nondisplaced fractures of the anterior and posterior tables rarely require operative intervention. Displaced fractures of the anterior table cause a depression in the forehead and are usually elevated to correct forehead contour. If a nasofrontal duct is disrupted by a fracture, the frontal sinus is defunctionalized by removing all mucosa and obliterating it with bone graft. Displaced fractures of the posterior table are treated by "cranialization" of the frontal sinus. The posterior wall of the frontal sinus is removed, its ducts plugged, and a pericranial flap is placed over the defect such that the former sinus becomes part of the intracranial contents.

Orbital Fractures

The paired orbits are modified pyramids formed by seven facial bones that contain the globes, extraocular muscles, orbital fat, and nerves. The thick bone of the orbital rim and lateral orbital wall contrasts with the paper thin bone of the medial and inferior walls. Signs and symptoms of orbital fractures include diplopia, visual changes (caused by optic nerve pathology), enophthalmos, exophthalmos, vertical dystopia, cheek numbness (due to injury to the infraorbital nerve which runs in a groove in the orbital floor), globe abnormalities, periorbital lacerations or bruising, and palpebral or subconjunctival hematomas. Thorough ophthalmological examination for visual acuity, visual field deficits, globe rupture, retinal detachment, and hyphema is performed. Also, a forced duction test, in which the insertion of the inferior rectus muscle on the globe is forcibly moved to rule out entrapment, is performed in all patients with diplopia. A facial CT scan aids in confirming the diagnosis.

Nondisplaced orbital fractures can be managed with observation. Displaced orbital fractures leading to entrapment or volume increase are explored in the operating room. The usual surgical approaches are either the transconjunctival or subciliary. Orbital rim fractures are reduced and fixated with titanium plates and screws. Orbital wall fractures are treated by reducing the orbital contents and placing alloplastic sheets (Medpor, Supermid), bone graft, or titanium mesh in position to maintain orbital volume. In the early postoperative period, it is important to monitor optic nerve function because blindness is a risk of surgery.

Nasal Bone Fractures

The prominent nasal bones are the most commonly fractured facial bones. Patients with nasal bone fractures commonly present with pain, swelling, nasal deviation, and epistaxis. In addition to examination of the external nose, a nasal speculum is inserted into the nose to evaluate the nasal septum. Septal hematomas require immediate drainage to avoid septal necrosis.

Most nasal bone fractures can be managed by closed reduction techniques and splinting. Late deformities such as a dorsal hump, saddle-nose deformity, and deviation can be managed with formal rhinoplasty (see Chapter 10).

Naso-Orbito-Ethmoidal Fractures

Fractures of the naso-orbito-ethmoidal complex of the central midface have a high potential for significant facial deformity because of displacement of the nose and eyes. Injury leads to lateralization of the frontal processes of the maxilla, which in turn leads to widening of the intercanthal distance, or telecanthus. Other common stigmata include a wide and shortened nose, epistaxis, orbital hematomas, and crepitance over the involved area. The frontal processes of the maxilla are mobile on palpation. Examination of the lacrimal apparatus, including the nasolacrimal duct, reveals concomitant injury.

Naso-orbito-ethmoidal complex fractures demand open reduction and internal fixation to relieve telecanthus and nasal deformities. If injured, the lacrimal duct may be repaired with fine suture and stented with silastic tubing.

Zygomatic Fractures

Because of the prominence of the cheek, the zygoma (cheek bone) is commonly fractured. The zygoma articulates with the maxilla medially and inferiorly, the frontal bone superiorly, the sphenoid bone laterally, and the temporal bone via its arch. With the exception of isolated zygomatic arch fractures, all fractures of the zygoma affect the orbit, and thus diagnosis and treatment incorporates the orbit. Isolated zygomatic arch fractures are managed nonoperatively or through small incisions (the Gilles approach). Displaced fractures of the body of the zygoma with resultant orbital and cheek deformity are treated with open reduction and internal fixation.

Maxillary Fractures

Fractures of the maxilla essentially involve the entire midface region, and are classified by the Le Fort classification system. Le Fort fractures can occur unilaterally, bilaterally, in combination (a left Le Fort II and right Le Fort III), and at multiple levels (a left Le Fort I and III). A Le Fort I fracture is a transverse fracture separating the lower, tooth-bearing segment of the maxilla from the rest of the midface. A Le Fort II fracture is pyramidal in shape, and separates the tooth-bearing, lower maxillary bone from the orbits and upper craniofacial skeleton. A Le Fort III fracture, or craniofacial dysjunction, separates the upper maxilla from the skull base. The hallmark of a Le Fort fracture is mobility of the maxilla on physical examination. Other signs and symptoms include orbital hematomas, epistaxis, pain in the midface, facial elongation, midface retrusion, and tooth occlusal abnormalities.

Nondisplaced Le Fort fractures may be managed nonoperatively. Displaced Le Fort fractures often require open reduction and internal fixation, as well as maxillomandibular fixation. Important concerns include stabilization of tooth occlusion and reduction of facial buttresses.

Mandible Fractures

The prominent position of the mandible makes it the second most commonly fractured facial bone. Because of its shape, it is commonly broken in two places. Areas that are weakest, like the subcondylar area, are the most frequently fractured. A mandible fracture is suspected any time acute malocclusion exists in the trauma setting. Other signs and symptoms of a mandible fracture include pain, swelling, trismus (pain on moving the jaw), inability to open or close the jaw, fractured teeth, discrepancies in the height of dentition, and intraoral lacerations. Radiographic examination with a CT scan or **Panorex** aids in diagnosis. (A Panorex is a specialized plain radiograph in which the x-rays rotate around the mandible, essentially transforming it from a curved structure to a flat image.)

Treatment of mandible fractures always begins with restoration of occlusion. It is essential that all stable teeth are reduced to their premorbid location so that the patient can continue to chew food. Restoration of proper occlusion usually requires binding the maxillary and mandibular teeth together with a series of wires, screws, or arch bars, so-called maxillomandibular fixation (MMF). Sometimes MMF is all that is required to adequately treat a mandibular fracture.

Many mandibular fractures require open reduction and internal fixation. This can be performed through intraoral lower gingivobuccal sulcus incisions, extraoral incisions, or percutaneous methods. Titanium plates and screws hold the reduced bony segments in place. Complications of mandibular fracture treatment include chin numbness from injury to the inferior alveolar nerve, malocclusion, nonunion of bony segments, and infection.

Breast and Trunk Reconstruction

Nia D. Banks, MD, PhD

Breast Anatomy

Development of the female breast marks the beginning of puberty. In preparation for fulfilling its role as a lactating organ, the breast develops glandular architecture consisting of epithelial-lined lobules and ducts that converge at the nipple areolar complex (NAC). The anatomic borders of the breast include the second rib superiorly, the seventh rib inferiorly, the sternum medially, and the axilla laterally. The **tail of Spence** is the most superolateral extent of the breast. In the absence of ptosis, the nipple generally overlies the fourth intercostal space. The major supporting structures of the breast are the skin "brassiere" and Cooper's ligaments, suspensory ligaments connecting the pectoralis fascia underlying the breast parenchyma to the overlying dermis.

Blood supply to the breast is rich, originating from perforators of the internal mammary artery medially, the axillary artery superiorly, and intercostal artery perforators laterally. Venous drainage closely follows the arterial system. Lymph drains primarily to axillary lymph nodes, although as much as 15% of lymphatic drainage is filtered by internal mammary lymph nodes. Innervation includes lateral and anterior branches of intercostal nerves and supraclavicular branches of the cervical plexus. The **lateral cutaneous branch of the fourth intercostal nerve** travels within the pectoralis muscle before reaching the NAC. This nerve provides primary sensation to the NAC, although branches of the second, third, and fifth intercostal nerves contribute as well.

The breast continues to develop throughout puberty and enlarges during each pregnancy. Breast ptosis, or sagging, is a natural progression of the aging breast as it succumbs to the effects of gravity. Involution of duct tissue and replacement by adipose tissue is also a normal process of aging.

Breast Cancer

■ Epidemiology

The American Cancer Society documented 212,600 new cases of breast cancer and over 40,000 deaths from breast cancer in 2003. Lifetime risk is 11%, which means one in nine women in the United States will develop breast cancer in her lifetime. Breast cancer is the most common cancer and the second leading cause of cancer death among women, second only to lung cancer.

■ Risk Factors

Risk factors for breast cancer include female sex, advancing age, family history in a first-degree relative, personal history of breast cancer, early first menses, late menopause, nulliparity or late first pregnancy, lobular carcinoma *in situ* (LCIS), and atypical ductal hyperplasia.

Despite the importance of family history, the vast majority (80%) of breast cancers are sporadic; 15% of women with breast cancer have a family history and the remaining 5% have inherited a single mutation that leads to the development of breast cancer (BRCA1 and BRCA2 are well-studied examples). Women who carry the BRCA1 or BRCA2 mutation have an 85% cumulative lifetime risk for breast cancer. These women should have close surveillance consisting of *semiannual clinical examinations, monthly self-examinations beginning in their teens, and annual mammograms from age 25 to 35 or 10 years younger than the youngest affected family member*. Affected individuals also benefit from chemoprevention with tamoxifen, and many opt for prophylactic bilateral mastectomy.

■ Histopathology

Breast cancer can be broadly divided into epithelial tumors arising from cells lining ducts or lobules and nonepithelial tumors arising from supporting stroma. Over 90% of cancers are epithelial and include **ductal carcinoma *in situ* (DCIS)**, LCIS, **infiltrating ductal carcinoma**, and **invasive lobular carcinoma**. DCIS is the proliferation of malignant ductal epithelial cells contained within breast ducts without invasion of the basement membrane. DCIS is considered a premalignant lesion, although invasive ductal carcinoma is found in 10% to 20% of specimens and the risk for developing a subsequent invasive cancer is about 25% to 30%. LCIS is a proliferation of malignant epithelial cells contained within breast lobules without invasion of the basement membrane. LCIS is considered a marker for increased risk of development of invasive cancer because the risk for developing subsequent invasive cancer (usually ductal) in either breast is about 20%. LCIS tends to be bilateral and multicentric, with LCIS identified in 50% to 90% of contralateral breast specimens. Invasive ductal carcinoma accounts for greater than 75% of invasive breast cancer. Invasive lobular carcinoma makes up the remaining 8% to 10% of invasive epithelial breast cancer. Histologic types such as Paget's disease of the breast, inflammatory breast carcinoma, and sarcoma represent the remaining 5% to 10% of breast cancers.

Other prognostic indicators include nuclear and histologic grade, presence or absence of estrogen and progesterone receptors, DNA content, and overexpression of the *c-myc* and HER-2/*neu* protooncogenes. Clinical staging is more important than histology in determining prognosis.

■ Clinical Manifestations

Most breast cancers present as a palpable mass found by the patient on routine self-examination. They are typically firm, nontender, relatively immobile masses commonly found in the upper-outer quadrant of the breast. Bloody nipple discharge, skin dimpling, nipple inversion or retraction, and skin ulceration usually indicate malignancy. Dermal lymphatic invasion commonly seen in inflammatory breast cancer may give the skin a warm, edematous, erythematous appearance commonly termed *peau d'orange* (orange peel). Presence of axillary lymphadenopathy signifies metastatic spread to the axillary lymph nodes. Other signs of metastasis to lungs, liver, brain, and bone include weight loss, dyspnea, hemoptysis, cough, jaundice, headache, changes in vision, bony pain, and pathologic fractures.

■ Treatment and Prognosis

Breast cancer staging is determined by the TNM (tumor, node, metastasis) system and is meant to guide treatment and aid in determining prognosis (Table 7-1). Stage 0 disease includes DCIS and LCIS and is treated by wide local excision with tumor-free margins or simple mastectomy, since, by definition, these lesions are contained within the breast. Simple mastectomy refers to the removal of all breast tissue, NAC, and skin without performing an axillary node dissection. Patients with stage I and II disease are candidates for **modified radical mastectomy (MRM)** or **breast conservation therapy (BCT)**. The latter consists of lumpectomy, axillary lymph node dissection or sentinel lymph node biopsy, and subsequent radiation to reduce the risk of local recurrence. MRM includes the removal of all breast tissue, pectoralis fascia, NAC, skin, and axillary lymph nodes. Patients with stage III and IV cancer undergo multimodal treatment consisting of modified radical mastectomy,

▇ TABLE 7-1 Breast Cancer Staging, Treatment, and Prognosis

Stage	TNM	Surgical Treatment	Adjuvant Treatment	5-Year Disease-Free Survival
0	Tis (DCIS or LCIS), N0, M0	Local excision Simple mastectomy	None indicated	100%
I	T1 (tumor ≤ 2 cm), N0, M0	BCT MRM	±Tamoxifen or chemotherapy	85%
II	T1, N1 (ipsilateral axillary nodes), M0 T2 (2–5 cm), N0, N1, M0 T3 (>5 cm), N0, M0	BCT MRM	±Tamoxifen or chemotherapy Chemotherapy and/or tamoxifen for all N1	65%
III	T3, N1, M0 T4 (into chest wall), Any N, M0 Any T, N2 (matted axillary nodes), M0 Any T, N3 (internal mammary nodes), M0	MRM	Radiation Chemotherapy and/or tamoxifen	40%
IV	Any T, any N, M1 (distant metastases)	MRM	Radiation Chemotherapy Hormonal therapy	10%

BCT, breast conservation therapy; MRM, modified radical mastectomy; T, tumor size; N, nodal involvement; M, distant metastasis.

radiation therapy, and systemic chemotherapy with or without hormonal therapy. As stated previously, radiation therapy assists with local-regional control. Chemotherapy and hormonal therapy are indicated for adjuvant therapy for node-positive patients and high-risk node-negative patients, and as palliation for metastatic disease.

Breast Reconstruction

Breast reconstruction after mastectomy significantly improves a patient's concept of body image and can be an important part of the rehabilitation process. Options for breast reconstruction follow the reconstructive ladder (see Chapter 3) and include external prostheses, expanders/implants, and autologous tissue reconstruction using pedicled flaps and free tissue transfer. The method of reconstruction depends on quality of skin flaps and size of skin defect after mastectomy, size of the opposite breast, medical comorbidities that may preclude autologous tissue reconstruction, the patient's ability to tolerate a larger operation, patient preference, and body habitus. Timing of reconstruction depends on patient preference, tumor biology, and need for adjuvant therapy. Importantly, breast reconstruction does not interfere with future cancer surveillance, decrease disease-free survival, affect overall survival, or decrease time to recurrence. Furthermore, it does not interfere with the administration of adjuvant therapies.

■ External Prostheses

External prostheses have been used for centuries to camouflage mastectomy defects. Commonly made of foam rubber or silicone, they fit into the cup of a brassiere and look quite normal under clothing. They are the best option for patients who are not surgical candidates.

■ Expanders/Implants

Placement of a tissue expander or breast implant beneath the soft tissues of the chest wall provides a breast mound of acceptable volume and shape in women with small to moderate-sized breasts. The implant/expander can be placed beneath the mastectomy flaps or in the submuscular position, beneath the pectoralis major muscle. Many surgeons prefer submuscular placement because it decreases the risk for capsular contracture and softens contours of the reconstructed breast by interposing another layer of healthy autologous tissue between the implant and the skin. The most common complications of implant reconstruction are infection, implant rupture, capsular contracture, and ischemia/necrosis of mastectomy flaps.

■ Autologous Tissue Reconstruction—Pedicled Flaps

Pedicled Transverse Rectus Abdominis Myocutaneous Flap

The pedicled transverse rectus abdominis myocutaneous (TRAM) flap is the most commonly used source of autologous tissue for breast reconstruction (Figure 7-1). Its advantages include a large volume for creation of a large breast mound, a reliable muscle and skin "paddle," and an abdominoplasty, or tummy tuck, for the donor site.

The rectus abdominis muscle originates from the cartilage of the sixth, seventh, and eighth ribs, inserts onto the pubic tubercle

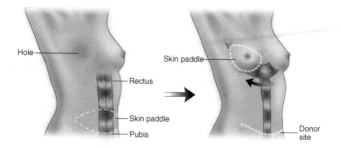

Figure 7-1 • Pedicled TRAM flap.

and pubic crest, and acts to flex the abdomen and provide domain for intraabdominal organs. The pedicled TRAM flap includes muscle from the rectus abdominis and a skin paddle from the lower abdomen. The flap receives blood supply from the superior epigastric artery and its perforating branches. The deep inferior epigastric artery (DIEA) is the rectus abdominis muscle's dominant pedicle, but the superior epigastric artery and vein can adequately support the flap in most cases.

Survival of a larger skin paddle is ensured by delaying or supercharging the flap. Delaying the flap refers to ligation of the deep inferior epigastric artery 2 weeks prior to flap harvest in order to allow the muscle/flap to acclimate to its altered perfusion. Supercharging the flap refers to connecting the DIEA into vessels in the axilla so that the flap has a dual blood supply. Complications from a pedicled TRAM flap include abdominal wall weakness, abdominal wall hernias, fat necrosis on the flap periphery, donor site seroma, and flap necrosis. Increased complications have been observed in patients with a pendulous abdominal panniculus, diabetes, history of tobacco use, and previous abdominal surgery that violated the rectus abdominis muscle.

Latissimus Dorsi Myocutaneous Flap

The latissimus dorsi muscle (LDM) originates from the spinous processes of T7–T12 and L1–L5, the sacrum, the posterior superior iliac crest, and ribs 9 through 12 and inserts anteriorly onto the proximal humerus. The LDM assists the pectoralis with shoulder adduction and extension (e.g., when using the arms to climb). It is a **Mathes and Nahai type V muscle** with one dominant pedicle entering the lateral edge of the muscle and several segmental pedicles based on medial perforators.

For breast reconstruction, the LDM is raised as a pedicled flap based on the dominant **thoracodorsal neurovascular bundle**. If the thoracodorsal artery was ligated or injured during the axillary dissection, the LDM can still be used if there is retrograde flow through the serratus branch of the artery. Care must also be taken to preserve the thoracodorsal nerve, because denervation will lead to atrophy of the muscular components of the flap.

The LDM has several advantages: it provides reliable vascularized muscle with or without skin, it is versatile and can be used with or without an implant/expander, it can be harvested as an extended latissimus dorsi myocutaneous flap (which includes soft tissue from the lower back to increase volume), and the donor site can be closed primarily. Limitations of this flap for breast reconstruction include inability to reconstruct a large breast without an implant and frequent donor site seromas and hypertrophic scarring.

■ Autologous Tissue Reconstruction—Free Tissue Transfer

Transverse Rectus Abdominis Myocutaneous Free Flap and Its Derivatives

The free TRAM was developed to minimize the major problems associated with the pedicled TRAM—partial flap loss due to marginal blood supply and abdominal wall weakness caused by harvesting a large portion of the rectus abdominis muscle. The free TRAM maximizes perfusion to the lower rectus abdominis musculocutaneous tissue by using the muscle's dominant pedicle, the DIEA, as its blood supply. It minimizes donor site morbidity by taking less muscle and fascia. In fact, the deep inferior epigastric artery perforator (DIEP) flap leaves all of the rectus abdominis muscle and fascia behind. The thoracodorsal artery in the axilla and the internal mammary artery (IMA) below the sternum are commonly used recipient vessels. The thoracodorsal artery is readily available and exposed if there has already been an axillary dissection and leaves the IMA as a potential graft for future coronary bypass surgery. On the other hand, the internal mammary artery is of larger caliber, providing superior flow and a technically easier anastomosis. Furthermore, using the IMA prevents lateral fullness that occurs when a flap is inset in the axilla.

Other sites commonly used for free tissue transfer to the breast include the superior gluteal artery perforator (S-GAP) flap, anterolateral thigh flap, and "Rubens" flap from excess fat over the iliac crest. Procedures on the contralateral breast—reduction, mastopexy, or implant augmentation—may also be required to enhance the aesthetic outcome.

■ Nipple Areolar Complex Reconstruction

The final stage of breast reconstruction involves creating a new nipple areolar complex and is done as a separate procedure to ensure proper location of the NAC on the new breast mound. Options for reconstruction include **tattooing**, **composite grafts from the contralateral nipple**, and **local tissue rearrangement** to reproduce nipple elevation. Tattooing has become increasingly popular both alone, and as an adjunct to local tissue rearrangement. Intradermal injection of pigment can be tailored to match the contralateral NAC in shape, size, and color. Contralateral grafts usually "take" well, but sacrifice elevation and volume of the preserved nipple. Many local flaps have been designed to mimic a nipple. The "skate" flap is popular, as it renders a nipple with reasonable volume and projection in addition to creating an areola.

Reduction Mammaplasty

■ Etiology

Macromastia is thought to result from an increased sensitivity to the trophic effects of estrogen on the breast, causing an increase of fibrous tissue and fat relative to glandular elements. Gigantomastia (virginal or juvenile hypertrophy) is an extreme form of macromastia that generally affects girls in early puberty.

■ Clinical Manifestations

Disproportionately large breasts can cause chronic headaches, back aches, neck and shoulder pain, or chronic irritation and infection of the inframammary fold. They can limit a woman's involvement in exercise and sports and be a source of anxiety, especially for adolescents. Women who suffer physically or psychologically from large breasts often benefit from bilateral reduction mammaplasty. Surgical breast reduction is best performed when breast growth is complete. That said, surgery may be indicated at a younger age when the benefits of normal psychosocial development outweigh the risks of surgery. A thorough preoperative breast examination and mammogram should be obtained for older patients and for younger patients with risk factors for breast cancer.

■ Treatment

The goals of reduction mammaplasty are to relieve symptoms, remove excess breast tissue and skin, minimize scar, and reposition the nipple areolar complex so that it resides at or above the level of the inframammary fold. All this must be accomplished while preserving lactation and sensation to the NAC. This generally involves excising skin from the lower quadrants of the breast, excising breast parenchyma from both lower and upper quadrants, and elevating the NAC with a dermoglandular bridge to maintain blood supply and innervation. The designs of the dermoglandular bridge and skin flaps are the main differences between techniques.

The Wise pattern and McKissock techniques use an inferior dermoglandular pedicle with skin from the upper breast. The vertical reduction mammaplasty avoids major scars along the inframammary fold, while the Passot technique avoids vertically oriented scars. Regardless of which technique is used, the patient should be measured and marked preoperatively in a standing or sitting position with a focus on position of the inframammary fold and NAC.

Specimens are identified by breast and quandrant in the event that an incidental cancer is found by pathology. Lateral dissection near the pectoralis major is limited to protect nipple innervation. Finally, the flaps are closed in multiple layers to minimize tension on the skin and drains are placed to minimize the risk for developing a seroma.

In extremely large reductions, the NAC is explanted from the amputated breast tissue and transferred as a free graft to the reformed breast mound. Free nipple grafts also reduce the length of the procedure and resultant blood loss and can be considered for patients who are elderly or who have significant medical comorbidities. Suction lipectomy can be used as an adjunct to further contour the reduced breast.

■ Follow-Up

Patient satisfaction after reduction mammaplasty is among the highest of all plastic surgery procedures. Even in the early postoperative period, patients have reduced symptoms, a more proportionate figure, and less limitation in physical activity.

■ Complications

Complications include loss of nipple sensation or erectile function, reduced ability to breast-feed, unsightly scars, wound infection, and recurrence. These risks must be weighed against the benefit of reduction for all patients, especially pubertal females. There is controversy as to whether scarring and fat necrosis after breast reduction can lead to mammographic abnormalities that would obscure or confuse the diagnosis of breast cancer. For this reason, many surgeons recommend reference mammograms before and after surgery and a low threshold for biopsy of suspicious lesions.

Mastopexy

■ Diagnosis

Mastopexy, or breast lift, repositions the nipple areolar complex to lie in its original, youthful position above the level of the inframammary fold, resuspends the skin "brassiere," and counteracts the sagging, or ptosis, caused by gravity over time. This natural aging process may be accelerated by weight loss, pregnancy and lactation, and menopause. Additionally, ptosis and flaccidity may be accompanied by unsightly striae. Breast ptosis is graded based on the relation of the NAC to the inframammary fold.

1. **First degree**—mild ptosis, nipple lies at the inframammary fold.
2. **Second degree**—moderate ptosis, nipple lies below the fold but above the most projecting portion of the breast.
3. **Third degree**—severe ptosis, nipple lies at the lowest contour of the breast.
4. **Pseudoptosis**—inferior pole of the breast sags, leading to an increased areola-to-inframammary fold distance, but the NAC still lies above the level of the inframammary fold.

■ Treatment

Breast lift techniques are designed to reposition the NAC, improve glandular support, and tighten the skin brassiere with minimal scarring. Most patterns for mastopexy mimic those for breast reduction. That said, the patient seeking breast reduction seeks relief from pain and distortion, whereas the patient seeking mastopexy desires aesthetic improvement. Thus, pattern and scarring are less well tolerated, which has led to the development of techniques based on minimal scar. Rather than dermolipectomy, tissue is saved and manipulated to improve breast projection. With mild ptosis and pseudoptosis, a good result can be achieved by simply augmenting the breast with an implant or by excising excess skin around the areola (a crescent or donut mastopexy). With more advanced ptosis or in patients that do not desire augmentation, a more extensive skin excision is required.

As the degree of ptosis increases, the distance the NAC must be moved and the amount of skin redundancy increases. Larger skin excisions can be accommodated by extending a circumareolar excision vertically or obliquely (vertical scar technique).

For larger excisions still, a horizontal component is added at the inframammary fold at the inferior extent of the vertical scar (inverted T excision). A Benelli mastopexy uses strong nonabsorbable suture to form a purse-string at the edge dermis after the circumareolar excision of a donut mastopexy. In this technique, the same type of suture is used to pexy the inferior portion of the gland to the periosteum of the ribs above.

Augmentation Mammaplasty

Breast augmentation is becoming increasingly common. Around 1% of the female population has implants. Most women undergo breast augmentation to improve self-image or advance socially and economically, but it is a valuable tool in breast reconstruction as well. Variables in the augmentation equation include size of the implant, composition of the implant, type of incision, and the anatomic position of the implant pocket.

■ Size of Implant

Choosing the size of the implant is difficult, because bra cup sizes are relative rather than absolute. Various methods have been used to predict the appropriate implant size, including placing a proposed implant inside a patient's bra and making volumetric predictions based on a patient's existing chest wall measurements. As a general rule, each 100 mL of implant volume will increase the size of the breast by one cup size.

■ Shell Characteristics

Implant shells can be smooth or textured. Textured implants prevent movement of the implant and prevent linear deposition of collagen, thus decreasing the rate of capsular contracture.

Implants can be round or "anatomic" (shaped like a teardrop). Anatomic implants help maintain lower pole fullness for patients who desire greater projection.

■ Composition

Implants are composed of a silicone shell filled with silicone gel or saline. Silicone gel–filled implants provide a reliable, durable result with a consistency that closely approximates that of a normal breast. Silicone gel–filled implants were used extensively in the United States prior to 1992, when the FDA prohibited their use due to anecdotal evidence linking them to autoimmune disorders. In 2003, a panel of experts gave testimony to the FDA refuting this link, however the FDA declined to accept the panel's recommendations to liberalize use of silicone gel–filled implants. Currently, silicone gel–filled implants are available in the United States only through FDA-approved clinical trials. They are still the preferred implant in Europe.

Saline implants have higher rates of deflation and capsular contracture, both of which predispose them to increased visibility. Smooth shell saline implants demonstrate visible rippling when slightly deflated. For these reasons, many surgeons consider saline implants to be inferior to silicone gel-filled implants.

■ Choice of Incision

The choice of incision for implant placement is a balance between exposure of the surgical site and a well-hidden scar. The inframammary fold incision was the first to be described, and it is still the most widely used. Other incisions include the periareolar, the transaxillary, the transareolar, and the transumbilical.

■ The Implant Pocket

Implants are placed on the anterior chest wall in a subcutaneous (prepectoral) or subpectoral position. Subcutaneous implants have better projection and less breast ptosis, but must be adequately covered by at least 2 cm of native soft tissue. Patients complain of less postoperative pain, and there is a shorter recovery period.

Subpectoral implants have better preservation of nipple sensation, a lower incidence of capsular contracture, and improved breast contour in thin patients. The subpectoral position allows for more accurate reading of mammograms, so it is the preferred method for women with risk factors for breast cancer.

■ Complications

Minor complications like hematoma, seroma, nipple hypesthesia, and hypertrophic scarring occur less than 5% of the time. Infection is rare but devastating, because the implant usually has to be removed. Theoretically, breast implants should not preclude breast-feeding because the glandular elements are not disrupted. However, there is a lower incidence of breast-feeding among women who have implants. Implants are not associated with higher rates of breast cancer or autoimmune disease. There is debate as to whether implants obscure breast cancer screening, and a routine screening mammogram is recommended before and after surgery for women with risk factors.

Complications related to the implants themselves include extrusion, rupture, and capsular contracture. Implant extrusion is exceedingly rare. The risk for rupture is about 2% per year. The periprosthetic capsule, the body's normal response to a foreign body, can hypertrophy, causing pain and abnormally shaped breasts. Treatment of capsular contracture requires open capsulotomy or capsulectomy (partial vs. total).

Gynecomastia

■ Etiology

Gynecomastia is an increase in male breast volume caused by fluctuations in male hormones. It occurs normally and transiently in newborns and during puberty due to a physiologically appropriate increase in estrogen exposure. The incidence in teenage boys is as high as 60%; the incidence rises again in older men to as high as 30%. The condition can be a normal variant, though it may be associated with more serious diseases. The common causes are an increase in estrogens, a decrease in androgens, or a deficit in androgen receptors. Thus, garden variety gynecomastia must be differentiated from breast cancer in a male breast, entities that impair degradation of estrogen, endocrinopathy, and inherited disorders.

■ Diagnosis

The diagnosis is largely based on history and physical examination. It is crucial to rule out medications, drugs, or illness as a cause of gynecomastia. Pharmacologic gynecomastia can be caused by cimetidine, digoxin, diazepam, exogenous estrogen, marijuana, reserpine, spironolactone, or theophylline. Secondary gynecomastia results from hormone-producing tumors (testicular, adrenal, pituitary, or lung), hypogonadism, liver disease, malnutrition, Klinefelter's syndrome, renal disease, or hypo-/ hyperthyroidism. Persistent gynecomastia in an adolescent boy (>18–24 months of age), tender or painful breasts, long-standing gynecomastia, or any breast tissue in patients at risk for breast cancer (men carrying the BRCA1 or 2 mutation and patients with Klinefelter's syndrome) are indications for surgery.

■ Treatment

Suction lipectomy has revolutionized the treatment of gynecomastia. Most cases of mild to moderate gynecomastia are managed with suction lipectomy, often under local anesthesia. Moderate gynecomastia often requires excision of breast tissue through a periareolar incision with adjunctive suction lipectomy to taper the resection. Moderate to large gynecomastia may require both skin resection and nipple repositioning. Severe gynecomastia requires amputation of excess skin and breast tissue with free nipple grafting.

Trunk Reconstruction

■ Chest Wall Reconstruction

The chest wall serves both structural and functional roles. It provides form to the torso, protection for the lungs and heart, and a framework to support the muscles of inspiration and expiration. Chest wall defects caused by trauma, tumors, infection, or congenital absence may require obliteration of thoracic dead space and skeletal stabilization if more than four ribs have been resected. When soft tissue alone is needed, muscle and myocutaneous flaps provide bulk, bony coverage, and healthy blood supply to an area. Due to proximity, size, and versatility, the pectoralis major, latissimus dorsi, and rectus abdominis flaps are most often used.

If skeletal stabilization is required, alloplastic materials like Teflon, Gore-Tex, Marlex-methyl methacrylate composite are used. If there is residual infection that precludes the introduction of foreign material, split rib grafts or large muscle flaps can also stabilize the chest wall and prevent flail segments.

■ Congenital Defects

Pectus excavatum (funnel chest) and **pectus carinatum** (pigeon chest) are common congenital deformities of the chest wall that account for over 90% of all chest wall abnormalities. Predominantly in males, they are thought to be caused by overgrowth of costal cartilages relative to the chest wall. If the overgrowth exerts a downward, inward force, pectus excavatum results. If the resultant force is outward, the overgrowth presents as pectus carinatum. Most affected children present with aesthetic concerns, though pectus excavatum may cause dyspnea on exertion, presumably from compression of the heart which limits cardiac filling during exercise. Traditionally, the repair of pectus excavatum involved resecting the costal cartilages, fracturing the sternum forward, and supporting the newly positioned sternum with bone wedges, metal bars, or wires. Currently, the minimally invasive Nuss procedure is used, wherein two small incisions are made along the lateral chest wall, a plane is dissected deep to the bony chest wall, and a rigid bar is placed to elevate the anterior thoracic cavity. The Nuss procedure has provided excellent results with minimal scarring and pain.

Poland's syndrome is thought to arise from sporadic vascular accidents during embryologic development, which lead to absence of the sternal head of the pectoralis muscle, hypoplasia of the breast or nipple, deficiency of subcutaneous fat and axillary hair, and anomalies of the costal cartilages and anterior rib ends.

Anomalies of the ipsilateral upper extremity, including brachy-syndactyly and extremity shortening, can also occur. Reconstruction focuses on restoring the contour of the chest by replacing the deficient or absent pectoralis with a latissimus dorsi muscle flap. Additionally, females with Poland's syndrome usually undergo breast reconstruction with submuscular implant and nipple areolar complex reconstruction using any of the previously mentioned methods.

■ Sternal Osteomyelitis

Median sternotomy is the standard approach for the majority of cardiac surgery. Infection of the sternum can spread to adjacent pericardium, coronary artery suture lines, and cardiac valves causing life-threatening illness. Historically, mortality rates from sternal infections were as high as 50%, but outcomes have been greatly improved by the use of broad-spectrum antibiotics and single-stage débridement with muscle flap coverage. Risk factors for infection or sternal dehiscence are diabetes or the use of both internal mammary arteries for bypass grafting, which creates sternal ischemia.

Mild sternal wound infections are treated by opening the sternal wound, minimal débridement, and intravenous antibiotics. Moderate and severe sternal infections require aggressive débridement of all involved soft tissue and bone followed by muscle flap coverage. The pectoralis major is the flap of choice. This flap is a Mathes and Nahai type V muscle (see Chapter 3) and can be raised based on either of two vascular pedicles: the dominant thoracoacromial pedicle laterally and the segmental parasternal perforators medially. When based laterally, it is advanced into the void left by the sternum; based medially, it is turned over on itself to fill the void. Both pectoralis muscles can be mobilized, providing a wide range of reconstructive configurations. The pectoralis muscles are hearty, and flap loss is rare.

Other flaps used in treating sternal osteomyelitis include the rectus abdominis, the latissimus dorsi, and the omentum.

■ Posterior Trunk Reconstruction

Many of the same principles of chest wall reconstruction can be applied to the coverage of back wounds. Coverage of defects of the back must be durable, allow stretch, and stand up to the pressure encountered with sitting and standing. In addition to infection, radiation, congenital defects, and neoplasm, back defects can also be caused by exposure of plates and screws placed by neurosurgical or orthopedic surgeons. In terms of available coverage, the back can be divided into thirds. Soft tissue defects in the upper third are covered by the trapezius muscle; the latissimus dorsi muscle covers the middle third; the gluteus maximus muscle covers the lower third. Small defects near the spine can also be covered by mobilizing the paraspinous muscles. Defects from spina bifida can usually be covered by wide mobilization and primary closure. Larger defects may require muscle flaps.

8 Hand and Upper Extremity

Subhro K. Sen, MD and Jesse A. Taylor, MD

Hands, and in particular opposable thumbs, have played a large role in human ascendancy to dominance over the animal kingdom. The ability to use our hands forms the basis of much social and economic interaction. Thus, functional and cosmetic deficits in the hands are devastating.

Anatomy

The hand is a stable bony construct with mobile joints, functional muscle-tendon units, and intact sensation with a supple skin covering. The engineering and anatomy are complex, and this brief description will be somewhat superficial. However, an introduction to the functional anatomy will give you some feeling for the clinical issues faced by hand surgeons.

■ Bones

The radius and ulna comprise the bony forearm, articulating with the humerus proximally and the carpus distally. The wrist, or carpus, contains eight carpal bones made up of two rows of four bones each. From radial to ulnar, the proximal row consists of the scaphoid, lunate, triquetrum, and pisiform. The distal row consists of the trapezium, trapezoid, capitate, and hamate. The proximal row articulates with the ulna and radius. The distal row articulates with the five metacarpals, the bones of the palm of the hand. The heads of the metacarpal bones, which form the knuckles, articulate with the proximal phalanges. The thumb has two phalanges (proximal and distal); each of the other fingers has three (proximal, middle, and distal). The bones of the hand and wrist are held together by a complex system of ligaments.

■ Muscles

Extrinsic Flexors

Wrist flexors include the flexor carpi ulnaris (FCU) and the flexor carpi radialis (FCR). The eight tendons of the flexor digitorum superficialis (FDS) and profundus (FDP), the tendon of the flexor pollicis longus (FPL), and the median nerve pass through the carpal tunnel. The synovial and fibrous flexor sheaths cover the inner and outer surface of each tendon in the palm, respectively. The tendon of the FPL inserts onto the anterior surface of the base of the distal phalanx of the thumb. The tendons of the FDP course through the fibrosseous flexor tendon sheath to insert onto the volar surface of the bases of the distal phalanges. The tendons of the FDS split into two slips at the level of the shaft of the proximal phalanges to pass over the FDP tendon and insert onto the radial and ulnar sides of the middle phalanges. Although the fibrosseous flexor tendon sheaths are thick over the phalanges, they are attenuated over the joints.

Synovial sheaths cover the outer surfaces of the tendons to allow maximal glide and minimal friction. The synovial sheath of the FPL extends from the carpal tunnel to the distal phalanx. The common flexor synovial sheath (ulnar bursa) extends from the carpal tunnel to the palm of the hand. The digital synovial sheath to the small finger is contiguous with the ulnar bursa. The index, ring, and long fingers have separate digital synovial sheaths that extend from the metacarpophalangeal (MCP) joint to the insertion of the FDP tendons on the distal phalanges.

Extensors

The extensor tendons pass from the forearm, beneath the extensor retinaculum, and into the dorsum of the hand. The extensor retinaculum divides the extensor tendons into six compartments numbered from radial to ulnar.

1st compartment: abductor pollicis longus and extensor pollicis brevis
2nd compartment: extensor carpi radialis longus and brevis
3rd compartment: extensor pollicis longus
4th compartment: extensor digitorum and extensor indicis
5th compartment: extensor digiti minimi
6th compartment: extensor carpi ulnaris

Distal to the MCP joint, the extensor digitorum tendons broaden to form a highly specialized "extensor hood." This extensor expansion splits into three parts: a central slip that inserts on the base of the middle phalanx, and two lateral bands that converge to insert onto the base of the distal phalanx. The extensor indicis proprius and the extensor digiti minimi also join the extensor expansion of the index and small fingers, respectively.

The extensor carpi ulnaris (ECU) inserts onto the posterior side of the base of the fifth metacarpal to extend and ulnarly deviate the wrist. The abductor pollicis longus (APL) inserts onto the lateral side of the base of the first metacarpal bone to abduct the thumb. The extensor pollicis brevis (EPB) and longus (EPL) insert onto the dorsal base of the proximal phalanx and distal phalanx of the thumb, respectively, to extend the thumb. The extensor carpi radialis longus (ECRL) and brevis (ECRB) insert onto the base of the second and third metacarpal bones, respectively, to extend the wrist.

Intrinsic Muscles of the Hand

The four groups of intrinsic muscles are the lumbricals, interossei, thenar, and hypothenar. The palmarly based intrinsic muscles occupy the space between the metacarpals. The thenar and hypothenar compartments contain an abductor, an opponens, and a flexor muscle for the thumb and little finger, respectively.

The four lumbricals arise from adjacent sides of the tendons of the flexor digitorum superficialis and profundus to flex the MCP joints and extend the interphalangeal joints. Each lumbrical inserts onto the radial side of the base of the proximal phalanx of its corresponding finger. The lumbricals to the index and long fingers are innervated by the median nerve; the lumbricals to the ring and small fingers are innervated by the deep branch of the ulnar nerve.

There are four dorsal and three palmar interosseous muscles located in intervals between the metacarpal bones. All are innervated by the deep branch of the ulnar nerve. The first palmar interosseous muscle arises from the ulnar side of the base of the second metacarpal bone and inserts into the ulnar aspect of the index finger's proximal phalanx. The second and third originate from the radial aspect of the fourth and fifth metacarpals and insert onto the radial aspect of the proximal phalanges of the ring and small fingers, respectively. They adduct the fingers toward the hand's meridian. Additionally, they flex the MCP joints and extend the proximal interphalangeal (PIP) joints.

The dorsal interossei originate from the surface of adjacent metacarpals and insert onto the base of the proximal phalanges. The first and second insert onto the radial aspect of the index and long fingers, respectively. The third and fourth insert onto the ulnar aspect of the ring and small fingers, respectively. They act to abduct the fingers away from the meridian of the hand. Additionally, they flex the MCP joints and extend the PIP joints.

■ Arteries

The radial artery courses along the radial aspect of the volar forearm, passes dorsal to the tendon of the EPL, then passes palmarly between the two heads of the first dorsal interosseous muscle to form the deep palmar arch. The deep palmar arch joins with the deep palmar branch of the ulnar artery.

The ulnar artery descends on the radial border of the FCU muscle, passes over the flexor retinaculum on the ulnar side of the wrist, and enters the palm with the ulnar nerve via Guyon's canal. After giving off a deep palmar branch, it forms the superficial palmar arch, which is located between the palmar aponeurosis superficially and finger flexor tendons. Both the superficial and deep palmar arches connect under normal conditions so that the hand can survive off of blood supply by a single artery.

The patency of the palmar arches can be determined by Allen's test. Both arteries are occluded by manual pressure while the patient pumps the fist several times. Pressure is released from one artery, and capillary refill should be noted in the fingertips within 10 seconds. Failure to provide capillary refill in all fingers denotes vessel occlusion or incomplete arches.

■ Nerves

Radial Nerve

The radial nerve innervates the brachioradialis, anconeus, and ECRL proximal to the elbow, then divides into the sensory branch of the radial nerve and the posterior interosseous branch. The sensory branch of the radial nerve continues along the deep surface of the brachioradialis then surfaces just proximal to the radial styloid to pass to the dorsum of the hand to provide sensory feedback from the dorsum of the hand, thumb, index finger, long finger, and radial side of the ring finger to the level of the distal interphalangeal (DIP) joint.

The posterior interosseous nerve (PIN) pierces the fascia of the supinator muscle (the so-called "arcade of Frosche," which can cause nerve compression), then innervates the extensors of the wrist and hand. The last muscle to receive innervation from the PIN is the extensor indicis. Thus, it is useful to test the extensor indicis to differentiate partial and complete PIN injuries.

Median Nerve

The median nerve enters the forearm medial to the biceps tendon and lateral to the brachial artery. Near the elbow, it is next to the lacertus fibrosis and the pronator teres, both of which can cause nerve compression. As it courses distally, it assumes a position between the FDS and FDP, innervating all tendons of the FDS, the FPL, the pronator quadratus, and the index and long finger FDP. The palmar cutaneous branch of the median nerve exits just proximal to the carpal tunnel to provide sensory feedback from the base of the thenar eminence. The median nerve enters the hand via the carpal tunnel to supply the thenar muscles (abductor pollicis brevis, flexor pollicis brevis, opponens pollicis) and the radial two lumbrical muscles. Sensory fibers supply the palmar surface of the thumb, index finger, and long finger, and radial half of the ring finger (including their nail beds).

Ulnar Nerve

The ulnar nerve enters the forearm via the cubital tunnel, which is formed by the medial epicondyle and the medial wall of the olecranon. It passes deep to the two heads of the FCU, supplying motor innervation. It continues distally in the forearm deep and radial to the tendon of the FCU, giving off motor branches to the FDP to the ring and small fingers. Proximal to the wrist crease, the sensory branch of the ulnar nerve surfaces to provide sensory feedback from the small finger, ulnar half of the ring finger, and the ulnar border of the hand. The remainder of the ulnar nerve enters the hand via Guyon's canal to innervate the hypothenar muscles (abductor digiti minimi, flexor digiti minimi, opponens digiti minimi), all the interossei, and the ulnar two lumbricals.

Hand Injuries

■ History

A complete history of a hand injury should include hand dominance, time of injury, mechanism of injury, environment, overall medical condition, medications and allergies, tetanus status, any previous injury or hand surgery, occupation, and hobbies. Most hand injuries are work-related injuries in otherwise healthy individuals.

■ Physical Examination

Vascular Assessment

Vascular assessment begins by observing the color and temperature of the affected extremity. Skin turgor and capillary refill are assessed in each digit. Pulses are palpated; if nonpalpable, they are assessed with Doppler ultrasonography. Comparison with the contralateral upper extremity can be helpful. Allen's test determines patency of the palmar arches.

Sensory Assessment

The radial, median, and ulnar nerves are assessed by their distributions described above. A pinprick determines a patient's ability to distinguish sharp from dull. Light touch can be measured with a cotton tip applicator. Two-point discrimination may be tested with a paperclip (normal two-point discrimination is 2–3 mm at the fingertip).

Motor Assessment

Inferences about motor function often can be made prior to initiating the physical examination. Normally there is a gentle cascade of digits with increasing flexion going from index to small finger. Disrupted flexor tendons leave a digit's extensor mechanism unopposed, and thus the finger lies in a position of relative extension. Similarly, when extensor tendons are cut, the resting posture is a position of flexion. Thus, tendon injuries interrupt the hand's normal cascade of digits.

Motor function is assessed by isolating various joints and testing the muscles that move them. For instance, the FDP is tested by isolating the DIP joint in extension and asking the patient to flex it. The FDS is tested by stabilizing all fingers in extension and asking a patient to flex at the PIP joint. The muscles of the thenar and hypothenar compartments are tested by opposing the thumb and small fingertips (this is a good test of median nerve function as well). Ulnar nerve function is tested by asking the patient to extend the fingers and spread them apart, a test of interosseous muscle function. The radial nerve is tested by asking a patient to extend the digits with the wrist in extension. EIP and EDM can be tested separately from the extensor digitorum by asking the patient to extend the index and small fingers in isolation. The ECRL and ECRB are intact if the patient can hold the wrist in extension while the examiner applies a flexion force.

Diagnostic Imaging

Fracture is suspected if hematoma, deformity, decreased range of motion, or persistent local tenderness follows any injury. Plain radiographs, at least two views at 90 degree angles, provide a baseline assessment and are usually all that is needed to adequately diagnose and treat a fracture. CT scans, in general, are more sensitive for fractures and dislocations. MRI has become the procedure of choice for soft tissue injuries, including ligamentous and musculotendinous disruptions. Ultrasonography can be helpful in localizing fluid collections or imaging vessels. Fluoroscopy in the form of a C-arm is used extensively in the operating room to assess adequacy of reduction and fixation of a fracture.

■ Treatment (Box 8-1)

Fractures and Dislocations

The goal in management of fractures and dislocations is to restore bony alignment to regain the maximum amount of motion and strength possible when the patient has finally healed. How that is achieved—whether with splint or cast immobilization, percutaneous K-wire fixation, or plate and screw fixation—has significant impact on long-term hand function. The hand surgeon must keep the soft tissues in mind, especially those tendons expected to glide over bones, when choosing the method of fixation. Length of immobility may also have a profound effect, because

---

■ BOX 8-1 Acute Management Tips

- Irrigate all wounds copiously; débride devitalized tissue conservatively.
- Control bleeding with pressure and extremity elevation. Never blindly clamp bleeding vessels. A tourniquet or inflated BP cuff may be used to control bleeding for examination and treatment.
- Administer tetanus prophylaxis and antibiotics as needed.
- Complete the sensory examination before administering local anesthesia.
- Splint all hand injuries in intrinsic position as soon as possible. Splinting will help to control pain and stabilize injuries while diagnostic imaging is performed.
- Extensor tendon injuries may be treated in the emergency room.
- All flexor tendon injuries, open fractures, nerve injuries, and vascular injuries causing hemorrhage not controllable by direct pressure are best managed in the operating room.

---

stiffness and adhesions that develop as a result of immobility may limit long-term function. Healed fractures and dislocations require aggressive physical therapy regimens to improve strength and range of motion.

Tendon Injuries

FLEXOR TENDON INJURIES

Flexor tendon injuries are repaired with four sutures (e.g., 4-0 braided nonabsorbable) through the core for strength, and a fine epitendinous suture (e.g., 5-0 monofilament, nonabsorbable) for alignment. Injuries are classified into five zones (Figure 8-1) for purposes of physician communication and comparison of outcomes. Zone I is at the DIP level, where the FDP inserts into the base of the distal phalanx. Most flexor tendon injuries at this level require reinserting the tendon onto bone. Zone II is from the MCP joint to the DIP joint of the fingers, the region of the fibrosseous flexor tendon sheath. Zone II used to be called "no man's land" because of poor outcomes, largely due to formation of adhesions between the tendons and the tendon sheath. Additionally, portions of the flexor tendon sheath, termed pulleys, which keep the flexor tendons from bowstringing, must be cut to provide access to tendons and repaired in order to avoid bowstringing. Zone II injuries remain challenging, but better outcomes are achieved with a sturdy repair and early, aggressive hand physical therapy.

Zone III extends from the distal aspect of the carpal tunnel to the MCP joint, an area that is relatively easy to access. Injuries in zone IV, the carpal tunnel, are rare because the transverse carpal ligament protects the tendons. Zone V includes the area proximal to the transverse carpal ligament. In the distal portion of zone V the tendons are discrete structures, but in the proximal portion of

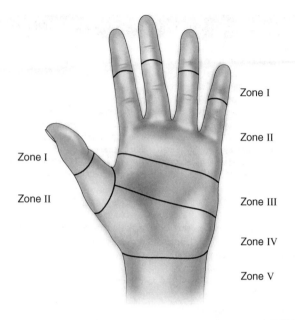

Figure 8-1 • Flexor tendon zones.

zone V there is the musculotendinous junction, which is a very poor site for repair because the tendons become thinner and fan out to join the muscle belly. Early, aggressive hand therapy is critical in maximizing long-term function.

EXTENSOR TENDON INJURIES

Extensor tendon injuries are repaired in a variety of ways based on the location of the injury. Proximally, where their shape mimics that of flexor tendons, repair is with four strong core sutures and a fine epitendinous suture. Distally, where they are flat bands, their ends are approximated with a single layer of interrupted stitches (e.g., 4-0 braided nonabsorbable). Extensor tendon injuries are classified into eight zones (Figure 8-2). Zone I is the area over the DIP joint and distal phalanx. Disruption of the tendon in zone I will cause **mallet finger**, where the DIP is slightly flexed at rest. Zone I injuries may be splinted if minimal; the tendon is reinserted into bone if there is complete transsection.

Zone II is the region over the middle phalanx of the digits and proximal phalanx of the thumb. Here the lateral bands of the extensor hood are frequently lacerated as they course toward their insertion. Primary repair with interrupted sutures is indicated if over 50% of the tendon is cut.

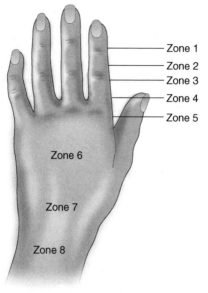

Zone 1
Zone 2
Zone 3
Zone 4
Zone 5
Zone 6
Zone 7
Zone 8

Zone of Extensor Tendon Injury

Figure 8-2 • Extensor tendon zones.

Zone III is over the PIP joint of the digits, where the central slip of the extensor hood inserts on the base of the middle phalanx and the MCP joint of the thumb where the extensor pollicis brevis inserts on the base of the proximal phalanx. Zone III injuries are treated by reinsertion of the central slip/EPB into the base of the corresponding phalanx, and centralization and repair of the lateral bands. Injuries in zone III can lead to a **boutonniere deformity** (PIP joint flexion and DIP extension) if the lateral bands slip volarly.

Zones IV and V correspond to the proximal phalanx and MCP joint, respectively. Repair is best performed with horizontal mattress sutures in a single layer. Injuries in Zones VI and VII on the dorsal hand are repaired with a four core and epitendinous repair. Zone VIII injuries in the distal forearm are treated similarly. Like flexor tendon repairs, all extensor tendon repairs require early, aggressive hand therapy to achieve maximal functional results.

Nerve Injury

Disrupted nerves are repaired primarily with fine (8-0), nonabsorbable suture. If tension-free coaptation cannot be achieved, a nerve graft (see Chapter 3) is used. When proper alignment of nerve fascicles is readily apparent, or if only a part of a nerve is lacerated, an epineural (outer covering of a nerve) repair may be used. When a nerve injury includes a crushing component or when there is a delayed repair, grouped fascicular repair is preferred. It is important to align motor and sensory fascicles by visual inspection when repairing large motor and sensory nerves such as the median and ulnar nerves. Epineural repair of severed digital sensory nerves is standard.

Amputation and Replantation

Initial management of an amputated part involves cleaning it, wrapping it in saline-moistened gauze, placing it in a plastic bag, and placing the plastic bag in ice water. Both the patient and the amputated part should undergo a standard physical and radiographic examination.

Children have an amazing capacity to heal, and virtually all amputated parts should be reattached regardless of circumstances. Considerations for replantation in adults include level of injury, location of injury, mechanism of injury, patient age, hand dominance, occupation, and suitability for rehabilitation. Relative contraindications include single digit amputations except for thumb, avulsion injuries with a large burden of devitalized tissue, previous injury to the amputated part, extreme contamination, warm ischemia time of over 6 hours, and advanced age. Most replanted parts make it out of the hospital alive, but long-term functional results depend largely on regaining sensation in the part, which takes months to assess. Range of motion in replanted joints is usually about half of normal, and most manual laborers require permanent job changes due to loss of dexterity. Best results are obtained with replantation of digits distal to the insertion of the FDS and hands at the wrist.

When replantation is not a consideration, treating an amputation involves débridement of devitalized tissue, shaping the remaining bone, burying any nervous tissue to avoid neuroma formation, obtaining hemostasis, and shaping soft tissue flaps to create a new fingertip. Patients usually recover rapidly from the surgery, and are back to work much more quickly than the replantation patients.

NERVE COMPRESSION SYNDROMES

Carpal Tunnel Syndrome

The carpal tunnel release is one of the most frequently performed operations in the United States. Carpal tunnel syndrome

(CTS) usually presents in the fifth and sixth decades of life, and the majority of patients are women. Just over half of patients with CTS present with bilateral symptoms.

The majority of cases are idiopathic, and are thought to be associated with overuse of the forearm and hand flexors. Patients with diabetes, thyroid disorders, amyloidosis, inflammatory arthritis, and alcoholism have higher rates of CTS. Masses or tumors in the region of the carpal tunnel may produce symptoms.

■ Clinical Manifestations

Typical symptoms are pain, paresthesia, hypesthesia, or numbness in the thumb, index finger, long finger, and radial aspect of the ring finger. Patients frequently complain of pain and numbness that awakens them from sleep in the middle of the night. Activities that require prolonged wrist flexion or gripping (driving a car, typing) may aggravate symptoms. Resting or splinting the forearm usually causes symptoms to subside.

On examination, the patient has numbness in the median nerve distribution of the hand. A positive **Tinel's sign**, which is a painful sensation of the fingers induced by percussion of the median nerve at the level of the palmar wrist, indicates regenerating median nerve fibers, a sign associated with CTS. **Phalen's test**, in which both wrists in a flexed position reproduces symptoms of CTS, is also sensitive for CTS.

■ Diagnostic Tests

The gold standard for diagnosing CTS is electromyography (EMG) and nerve conduction velocity (NCV). On EMG, patients have decreased fibrillation potentials in the abductor pollicis brevis. NCV in the median nerve is decreased.

■ Treatment

Patients with mild CTS who have no thenar atrophy can be treated with conservative therapy, which includes a resting splint with the wrist in neutral position and NSAIDs. Steroid injections of the carpal tunnel may be effective. If EMG shows impaired conduction of the median nerve at the wrist, if symptoms do not improve with 6 weeks of conservative treatment, or if there is evidence of thenar muscle wasting, a carpal tunnel release is indicated. Carpal tunnel release consists of dividing the flexor retinaculum, a procedure that may be performed via open technique or endoscopically. Patients are usually splinted for a short period after surgery, and a brief period of postoperative hand physical therapy is the norm.

Cubital Tunnel Syndrome

Cubital tunnel syndrome, or compression of the ulnar nerve at the elbow, occurs in approximately 10% of adults, a small percentage of whom actively pursue treatment. Those with a history of trauma to the medial aspect of the elbow are at risk for developing cubital tunnel syndrome.

■ Clinical Manifestations

Numbness in the ulnar hand is the chief complaint. Some patients notice an increased frequency of dropping objects from within their grip as well. A positive **Tinel's sign** is present over the ulnar nerve at the elbow. Patients also have a positive **Froment's sign**, a hyperflexed thumb interphalangeal joint when the thumb is pinching against the side of the base of the index finger (normally the interphalangeal joint is extended to provide maximal pinch). This is a sign of ulnar nerve palsy, because a lack of pinch power by the adductor pollicis (innervated by the ulnar nerve) is compensated for by the FPL.

■ Diagnostic Tests

As with CTS, EMG and NCV are the gold standard for diagnosing cubital tunnel syndrome.

■ Treatment

Mild cases are treated with nocturnal splinting to prevent extreme elbow flexion. Symptomatic patients with positive EMG/NCV require ulnar nerve decompression. Ulnar nerve decompression is accomplished by releasing the ligament of the cubital tunnel, medial epicondylectomy, subcutaneous ulnar nerve transposition, or submuscular ulnar nerve transposition. Postoperatively, patients are splinted for a week and undergo a short course of physical therapy thereafter.

HAND INFECTIONS

The most common cause of hand infections is trauma. Other predisposing conditions include diabetes and other neuropathic conditions. Ninety percent of infections are caused by gram-positive organisms: *Staphylococcus aureus*, *Streptococcus viridans*, group A *Streptococcus*, and *Staphylococcus epidermidis*. All hand infections require elevation and splinting of the affected extremity in addition to other therapies described below.

Infected Paronychia

An infected paronychia is an abscess of the soft tissue around the base of the fingernail. Patients typically present with pain, redness, and swelling at the base of the fingernail, which can be localized to one side of the nail, or diffuse, involving the entire paronychia. Treatment consists of incision and drainage of all pus, partial or complete nail removal, and twice daily cleansing of the affected digit until the wound is healed. Cultures usually grow *S. aureus*, for which an oral cephalosporin may be given.

Chronic paronychial infection may occur in individuals who immerse their hands in water throughout the day, like dishwashers. Cultures typically grow *Candida albicans*, and incision, drainage, and an oral antifungal are usually effective in treating the condition. Recurrent cases may require marsupialization (creation of an open pouch) of the paronychia.

Felon

A felon is an abscess of the volar pulp of the finger. Patients usually have a history of a puncture wound 5 to 7 days prior to the onset of symptoms. Extreme pain, redness, and swelling ensue. Treatment consists of draining the abscess, local wound care, and an oral cephalosporin. Cultures typically grow *S. aureus*. Severe felons cause necrosis of bone and soft tissues of the distal phalanx, requiring amputation and intravenous antibiotics.

Flexor Tenosynovitis

This painful infection of the tendon sheath and its contents presents with fusiform swelling of the finger, tenderness over the flexor tendon sheath, and pain on passive extension. The finger is usually held in slight flexion. Drainage of the infected synovial fluid (which can be purulent) is a surgical emergency. Delay in treatment may lead to loss of tendon function.

Bites

Human bites infect the hand most commonly with *S. aureus*, but also with *Eikenella corrodens* in a high percentage of clenched fist "fight bites." Resultant cellulitis may occur at any area of inoculation, but the classic fight bite occurs over the dorsal aspect of the MCP joint. Patients often present with a small laceration over the MCP (which has already closed by secondary intention), spreading redness around the laceration, and extreme pain with joint movement. Treatment of these penetrating injuries includes joint exploration, débridement, and irrigation. Multiple trips to the operating room for reexploration may be required to adequately treat the infection. Broad-spectrum intravenous antibiotics are administered as well.

Domestic animal bites and scratches commonly cause cellulitis, which can be treated with an oral penicillin on an outpatient basis. Deep puncture wounds demand attention similar to those of human bites, especially when they occur over a joint.

HAND TUMORS

Hand tumors vary from benign growths to malignant soft tissue tumors. Diagnosis is usually made from the history and physical examination, although radiographs and even tissue biopsy may be required.

The vast majority of tumors on the hand are benign. The most common are ganglion cysts, mucous cysts, giant cell tumor of the tendon sheath, epidermal inclusion cysts, and lipomas. The majority of these tumors can be left alone or treated by excision.

Vascular malformations can also occur in the hand. Lesions that are stable and asymptomatic are observed; those that progressively enlarge should be removed. Excision must be carefully planned around critical structures. Often a debulking procedure is enough to control the symptoms of the tumor.

Malignant bone tumors are commonly worked up with a CT scan and biopsy prior to definitive treatment. Malignant soft tissue tumors are best imaged with MRI. Resection is a common treatment modality, leaving patients with large functional and cosmetic deficits.

CONGENITAL ANOMALIES

The degree of deformity varies from minor, such as a digital disproportion, to severe, such as total absence of a bone. The Swanson classification of congenital hand anomalies groups deformities into broad categories:

1. **Failure of formation of parts.** This arrest in development causes complete absence of a part of the hand or upper extremity. Surgery is usually not performed, and these children are introduced to prosthetic devices early in childhood. Radial club hand, a deformity that involves all of the tissues on the radial side of the forearm and hand, is an example of failure of formation of parts.

2. **Failure of separation of parts.** With this type of deformity, parts of the hand and upper extremity fail to separate, a good example of which is syndactyly, or fusion of digits. Syndactyly is the most common congenital hand deformity, occurring in 7 of every 10,000 live births. It usually involves both hands, and males are more often affected than females. Complex syndactyly involves both bony and soft tissue fusion. Simple syndactyly implies only soft tissue involvement.

3. **Duplications of parts.** Duplication of digits is also known as polydactyly. The small finger is most commonly affected.

4. **Overgrowth of parts.** Overgrowth of parts is extremely rare. It is more commonly seen in males, and usually affects the index finger. Surgical treatment is complex, and the outcomes often poor. Amputation of the enlarged digit may be best.

5. **Undergrowth of digits.** Underdeveloped fingers or thumbs are associated with many congenital hand deformities. Surgical treatment is not always required to correct these deformities. Underdeveloped fingers may include the following: small digits, missing muscles, underdeveloped or missing bones, or absence of a digit.

6. **Congenital constriction band syndrome.** Thickened amniotic bands may wrap around an extremity *in utero* and cause ischemia or necrosis. Bands that form around an arm or a digit may cause hypoplasia distal to the constriction. If bands cause necrosis, children may be born without an extremity or digit.

Lower Extremity and Genitalia

Marwan Khalifeh, MD

LOWER EXTREMITY RECONSTRUCTION

The goal of lower extremity reconstruction is to salvage a threatened limb that will be more functional than a prosthesis following amputation. Over the past several decades, advances in rearrangement and transfer of soft tissues combined with advances in bone fixation and regeneration have provided reconstructive surgeons with many options. Lower extremity reconstruction remains a challenge, because our current options leave patients with lengthy recovery periods and abnormal ambulation. This chapter focuses on the traumatized patient, although the principles also apply to injury resulting from vascular disease, diabetes, or cancer.

Anatomy

A comprehensive review of lower extremity anatomy is beyond the scope of this chapter but several points are worth reviewing. The common femoral artery (CFA), a continuation of the external iliac artery, provides the main vascular supply to the extremity. In the proximal thigh, the CFA bifurcates into the profunda femoral artery, which supplies muscles in the thigh, and the superficial femoral artery (SFA). At the knee, the SFA becomes the popliteal artery, which trifurcates into the anterior tibial artery (which continues as the dorsalis pedis artery in the foot), the posterior tibial artery, and the peroneal artery. At least one of these three arteries is required for a viable foot. The venous system of the leg is divided into the superficial and deep systems. The deep system generally mirrors the arterial anatomy. The superficial system consists of the greater and lesser saphenous veins. Preservation of veins during débridement is a goal in order to avoid venous insufficiency.

Two nerves are necessary for lower extremity function: the **femoral nerve**, which is responsible for knee extension to facilitate ambulation, and the **tibial nerve**, which provides sensation to the sole of the foot. Damage to the tibial nerve is a relative contraindication to leg salvage in the adult patient, although nerves can be repaired in adults with varying success.

There are four muscle compartments in the lower leg: the anterior compartment, the lateral compartment, and the superficial and deep posterior compartments. The muscles of the lower leg are responsible for ankle movement, but ambulation with a fused ankle is possible, and loss of one or more of the muscular compartments is not a contraindication to leg salvage.

The skeletal anatomy of the lower extremity consists of the femur in the thigh and the tibia and fibula in the leg. The tibia supports more than 80% of the body's weight. It is prone to injury during trauma because it is protected only by skin and subcutaneous tissue. The fibula, on the other hand, is expendable except for its distal third, which is important for ankle stability.

Early Management

Common mechanisms of lower extremity trauma are motor vehicle accidents, gunshot wounds, and falls. The amount of energy transferred differs significantly between these types of injuries—motor vehicle collisions transfer 50 times the amount of energy of a bullet, which in turn transfers 20 times the amount of energy of a typical fall. Because tissue damage is proportional to energy transferred, wounds that appear similar on presentation progress differently when the mechanism of injury is different. The area of injured soft tissue, apparent or not, is termed the zone of injury.

All trauma patients are treated according to the principles of advanced trauma life support protocols, and injured limbs are addressed only after the patient is stabilized. In unstable patients, an amputation may be the safest course of action. After stabilization, a multidisciplinary team of plastic, orthopedic, and vascular surgeons assess whether a limb can be salvaged. Often a decision is deferred until the zone of injury demarcates.

■ Indications for Limb Salvage Surgery

Limb salvage is indicated when options for repair would make a patient at least as functional as an amputation and prosthesis at the level of injury. The salvaged limb should provide an acceptable degree of function and be pain free and durable enough to withstand the demands of normal daily activities. There are no absolute contraindications to limb salvage except critical illness precluding an operation. Several relative contraindications are included in Box 9-1.

■ **BOX 9-1 Relative Contraindications to Limb Salvage**

Systemic disease (diabetes, CHF, etc.)
Multisystem injury
Crush injury
Gustilo type IIIC injuries (vascular compromise)
Warm ischemia time >6 hr
Multiple level injury to the extremity
Disruption of tibial nerve in adults
Age >55 yr

■ **TABLE 9-1 Gustilo Fracture Classification**

Type I	Fracture with a clean cutaneous wound <1 cm in length
Type II	Fracture with laceration >1 cm in length lacking any severe soft tissue damage
Type III	Fracture with extensive soft tissue loss
	A Adequate coverage of the fracture by soft tissue despite extensive cutaneous lacerations or flaps; high-energy trauma irrespective of wound size
	B More extensive injury and contamination to the soft tissue, periosteal stripping and soft tissue gaps are present
	C Any open fracture with arterial injury requiring repair

Diagnosis

In a cooperative patient, a neurologic examination is conducted focusing on the sensation of the dorsum and sole of the foot. A normal sensory examination indicates intact nerves. A neural deficit may be the result of reversible injury with maintenance of nerve continuity or a disruption of nerve continuity that may require surgical coaptation. The remainder of the examination is best performed under anesthesia or sedation in patients able to perceive pain. Vascularity is assessed focusing on color, turgor, and pulses. The bones are inspected for fracture (Table 9-1), and bone fragments are assessed for viability, which depends on the degree of stripping from soft tissues. The skin and muscle are assessed and débrided, although frequently the initial soft tissue injury is underestimated, requiring further débridement. For instance, soft tissue avulsion may lead to random pattern flaps that do not have enough blood supply to survive but initially appear viable.

Plastic surgeons are needed for reconstruction and soft tissue coverage of Gustilo type IIIB and IIIC fractures.

■ **Patient Education**

The decision to reconstruct or amputate an extremity is seldom made emergently. Patient participation in the decision-making process is critical, because extremity salvage is a long and complicated process that usually requires multiple operations and a commitment to physical rehabilitation. It is the duty of the reconstructive surgeon to provide honest facts regarding the length of time and amount of work required on the part of the patient. Additionally, alternatives to reconstruction should be discussed fully. Amputation remains a good and sometimes preferable option, with faster time to ambulation, earlier return to work, and fewer operations. In a recent multicenter study, there was no difference in quality of life between patients with limb salvage and below-the-knee amputation. However, when given a choice, most patients prefer limb salvage to an amputation and prosthesis.

■ **Radiologic Evaluation**

Plain x-rays of the injured extremity are obtained on admission as part of the secondary survey. Traditional angiography delineates vascular anatomy best and can be obtained in the operating room when there is doubt about vascular patency. When planning a free tissue transfer, it is helpful to have an angiogram or a CT angiogram to assist with donor vessel selection. MRI is the preferred modality for diagnosing lower extremity osteomyelitis.

Treatment

■ **Skeletal Fixation**

Rigid skeletal fixation is the first step in limb salvage. The techniques available for fixation include intramedullary rod fixation, internal fixation with plates and screws, or external fixation (applying external "scaffolding" to the leg in order to keep bones in place). External pins can also be used with the Ilizarov technique for bone regeneration. In Gustilo type IIIB and IIIC fractures, external fixation is most commonly used because it destroys less of the blood flow to the bone, does not require immediate soft tissue coverage, and allows access to the wound for further débridement. Disadvantages of external fixation are pin tract infections, longer time to weight bearing than with internal fixation, and hindrance of access for microsurgery.

■ **Serial Débridement**

Adequate débridement of devitalized soft tissues and bone is an absolute requirement. Early débridement is associated with a decrease in wound infections and osteomyelitis. A balance must be achieved between adequate débridement and sacrifice of muscle groups, bone length, skin, and vessels. Attempts at preserving fracture fragments as bone grafts to avoid large bone defects are typically ill fated. Serial débridements at 2- to 3-day intervals are common, with the soft tissue defect being covered in the interim by either wet to dry dressings or a vacuum-assisted closure device. Once the wound is deemed clean and stable without further progression of necrosis, soft tissue coverage can proceed.

■ Skeletal Reconstruction

There are four primary methods for closure of bone gaps:

1. **Elimination** by shortening the limb and approximating the proximal and distal segments. A prosthetic shoe can be used for ensuing limb length deformity.
2. For bone gaps less than 7 cm, **bone grafting** 2 to 3 months after wound coverage is a good option, with bony union rates of greater than 90%. Methyl-methacrylate beads mixed with antibiotics can serve as space savers.
3. For defects greater than 7 cm, a **free bone flap** can be used. The fibula free flap, iliac crest, or scapula are appropriate donor sites.
4. **Distraction osteogenesis** involves disrupting the bony cortex at a site away from the site of injured bone and applying a force in the direction away from the corticotomy so as to lengthen the bone. Bone is created at a rate of approximately 1 mm/day, thus the bone gap is closed by 1 mm/day. The time to bony union is a long process, typically on the order of 6 months to a year.

Soft Tissue Management

■ Soft Tissue Coverage in the Thigh

Classical flap territories of the lower extremity are highlighted in Figure 9-1. Defects of the muscular thigh typically require simple advancement of local muscles to cover an exposed femur and a split-thickness skin graft to replace missing skin. Occasionally, a muscle flap is required to cover an exposed femoral artery or synthetic vascular graft or fill a hole created by an oncologic resection. The gracilis, sartorius, rectus femoris, or rectus abdominis muscle flaps are appropriate choices.

■ Soft Tissue Management of the Knee and Proximal Tibia: The Gastrocnemius Flap

Due to a paucity of local soft tissue, the knee and proximal tibia are two areas where muscle flaps are frequently required for

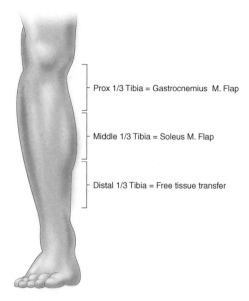

Prox 1/3 Tibia = Gastrocnemius M. Flap

Middle 1/3 Tibia = Soleus M. Flap

Distal 1/3 Tibia = Free tissue transfer

Figure 9-1 • Classic flap territories of the lower extremity.

bony coverage. The workhorse of soft tissue coverage around the knee and proximal tibia are the medial and lateral heads of the gastrocnemius muscle, which can fill a defect up to 9 cm medially and 5 to 7 cm laterally. One or both of these heads can be raised based on the lateral or medial sural arteries, which enter each muscle proximally from their tibial surface. The lesser saphenous vein and sural nerve travel in the cleft between the gastrocnemius muscles and should be preserved when possible. The function of the gastrocnemius is ankle plantar flexion as well as some knee flexion, but its loss is tolerable when the soleus muscle is preserved. Although muscles such as the tibialis anterior are in close proximity to the knee and proximal tibia, these muscles have a segmental blood supply (Mathes and Nahai type IV), cannot be mobilized extensively to cover the defect, and are often in the zone of injury (Figure 9-2).

■ Soft Tissue Management of the Middle Tibia: The Soleus Flap

The middle third of the tibia classically is covered by a soleus or hemisoleus muscle flap, which can cover defects of up to 10 cm in length. The vascular supply to the soleus is from the popliteal, posterior tibial, and peroneal vessels. The plantaris tendon, when present, lies between the soleus and gastrocnemius muscles. The

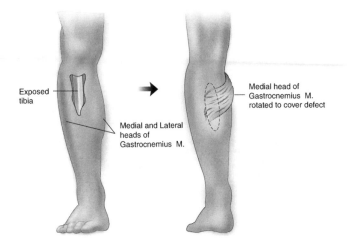

Exposed tibia

Medial and Lateral heads of Gastrocnemius M.

Medial head of Gastrocnemius M. rotated to cover defect

Figure 9-2 • Gastrocnemius muscle flap.

operation entails carefully dissecting the soleus muscle off the Achilles tendon and rotating it anteriorly. A hemisoleus flap can be raised, preserving the other half of the muscle for function. A split-thickness skin graft is typically needed for skin coverage.

■ Soft Tissue Management of the Distal Tibia and the Foot

Because there are no suitable muscle flaps that can be rotated to cover wounds in the distal tibia or the foot, free flaps are needed for exposed bone, joint, or tendon. Common flaps used are the latissimus, gracilis, and rectus abdominis muscles. Muscle flaps are thought to be especially valuable in providing well vascularized tissue and antibiotic delivery to devitalized beds, thereby decreasing the rate of infection. Fasciocutaneous free flaps such as the parascapular flap or anterior lateral thigh flap provide more durable coverage for sole of foot defects.

For injuries of the foot without massive soft tissue loss, local muscular and rotational skin flaps can be used. On the lateral aspect of the foot, the abductor digiti minimi muscle can be detached from its skeletal attachments and rotated based on the lateral plantar artery. The abductor hallucis brevis can be similarly mobilized on the medial aspect of the foot based on the medial plantar artery. Many local foot flaps have been described with mixed success. They minimize operative morbidity, and no bridges are burned if the flap fails.

■ Osteomyelitis

An all-too-common complication following treatment of open lower extremity fractures is the development of osteomyelitis. The use of prophylactic antibiotics in the perioperative period has been shown to decrease the incidence of osteomyelitis from 20% to 5%. Early débridement and soft tissue coverage of wounds has also been found to decrease the risk for osteomyelitis. Treatment of osteomyelitis consists of aggressive débridement of diseased bone followed by reconstruction of the bone and soft tissue defects.

GENITALIA RECONSTRUCTION

Penile Reconstruction

The development of the radial forearm flap has allowed reconstructive surgeons to reliably provide patients with an aesthetically acceptable and functional penis. The tubed radial forearm flap provides a neourethra, a reasonably sized tube, and durable skin that is usually a good color match. The vascular pedicle is the radial artery and cephalic vein. Coaptation of the pudendal nerves to the medial and lateral antebrachial cutaneous nerves can provide a sensate reconstruction. An implantable prosthesis can be inserted to mimic an erection.

Vaginal Reconstruction

Vaginal reconstruction can help minimize the sense of deformity associated with an oncologic resection. A tubed rectus abdominis myocutaneous flap, bilateral gracilis myocutaneous flaps, and bilateral fasciocutaneous flaps based on the internal pudendal arteries (so-called "Singapore" flaps) create acceptable neovaginas. Neovaginas are nonfunctional, but patients are able to have sexual intercourse.

10

Aesthetic Surgery

Jesse A. Taylor, MD

Aesthetic surgery is inherently different from other surgery in that the patient seeking an operation has no illness. Given the lack of pathology at the onset of an aesthetic consultation, the patient expects a smooth and uncomplicated operation and postoperative course. Most patients devote much time and effort into choosing their aesthetic surgeon. Additionally, the patient often selects the timing, anesthetic method, and even the surgical procedure itself. A competent surgeon develops rapport with the patient and helps to define realistic, achievable aesthetic goals. After planning an operation, it is important to educate patients on the risks inherent with anesthesia and surgery. Videotapes and instructional brochures can be helpful adjuncts.

Aging

Soft tissue ages because of three processes that interact over time: gravitational pull, sun exposure, and histologic changes within the skin and soft tissues. The relative contributions of these forces vary with different parts of the body.

Gravity affects all tissue layers, resulting in a lower position of the brow, hollowing of the infraorbital regions, more pronounced nasolabial folds, jowls, excess neck skin, abdominal wall laxity and pannus, and excess extremity skin and soft tissue.

The skin becomes thinner in all layers. Histologically, the epidermis changes the least, but there is a decrease in the number of melanocytes and Langerhans' cells. The dermis is most profoundly affected, with less ground substance, collagen, and elastin. All told, the aging process thins skin to 20% that of younger adults.

A lifetime of exposure to ultraviolet radiation from the sun leads to a classic leathery, wrinkled appearance. At the histologic level, sun-damaged skin is thicker, with thickened, damaged elastin fibers and an increased ratio of ground substance to mature collagen. Sun exposure also leads to DNA damage, altering the skin's ability to regenerate.

Finally, smoking leads to premature wrinkling, especially in the perioral region. It is thought that increased exposure to reactive oxygen species from cigarette smoke overloads the skin's antioxidant protective mechanism, leading to skin damage. Regardless, collagen synthesis is decreased by as much as 40% in chronic smokers.

Facial Proportions

Numerous studies have demonstrated ethnic and generational variation in normal values. The following information is intended to give students a general understanding of facial proportions recognizing that these generalities do not always hold true.

■ Face Height

The face can be divided into thirds of relatively equal height. The lower third extends from chin to the base of the nose and contains the mouth and lips. The middle third extends from the base of the nose to the root of the nose (termed the **nasion**). The upper third extends from the nasion to the hairline. The point from the hairline to the highest point on the head, the **vertex**, is approximately equal to another third of the facial height.

■ Forehead

The forehead is generally slightly less than a third of facial height. The normal male forehead has significant supraorbital bossing, or protuberance of the forehead just above the orbits. The mid-forehead is flat, and the upper forehead has a slight convex curvature to it. In contrast, the female forehead has little or no supraorbital bossing and more of a continuous mild curvature to it.

■ Brow

The eyebrow forms a gentle arch whose peak lies at the junction of the medial two thirds and lateral one third. This peak should lie midway between the lateral aspect of the iris and the lateral canthus of the eyelid. The brow should overlie the orbital rim in men and be several millimeters above the rim in women. The medial edge of the eyebrow should be in a vertical plane with the medial canthus of the eyelid and the lateral border of the nasal ala. The lateral edge of the eyebrow should lie slightly above the medial edge, and a line drawn between the lateral edge and the lateral edge of the nasal ala should touch the lateral canthus. The average distance between the upper edge of the eyebrow and the hairline is 5 cm; the average distance between the pupil and the upper edge of the eyebrow is 2.5 cm.

■ Eyes

The eyes are located at the junction of the middle and upper thirds of the face. They are separated by one eye breadth, which equals the width of the root of the nose. Average height of the bony orbit is about 19 mm measured at midorbit. The bony orbit is canted inferiorly such that the superior orbital rim generally lies 10 to 14 mm anterior to the inferior orbital rim.

The eyelids are distinguished by the medial and lateral canthi. The medial canthus is in line with a vertical plane taken from the lateral ala of the nose. The lateral canthus is approximately 3 mm cephalad to the medial canthus and usually about 3 cm lateral to it. The upper eyelid is larger, more curved, and much more active than the lower eyelid.

■ Ears

The external ear canal is located half the distance from the front of the face to the back of the head, and in a plane about midway between the eyes and the base of the nose. The ear protrudes from the skull at about a 20 degree angle, and the longitudinal axis of the ear usually lies 2 to 30 degrees posterior of the vertical axis.

■ Nose

The nose is a focal point in the face. Nasal height is generally two thirds midfacial height; nasal tip projection is approximately two thirds nasal height. Generally, the width of the base of the nose is approximately equal to the intercanthal distance. The dorsum of the nose projects 34 degrees from the face in women, 36 degrees from the face in men. The angle between the nasal base and the upper lip is 95 degrees in men and 110 degrees in women. In profile, a 2- to 3-mm wide segment of columella should be seen below the alar rims. The nostrils are oval and their long axes incline toward the nasal tip, giving the base a triangular shape.

■ Mouth, Lips, and Chin

The distance from the base of the nose to the inferior border of the upper lip is one third the height of the lower third of the face. The vermilion border of the lower lip is midway between the base of the nose and the chin. The corners of the mouth generally lie in a plane halfway between the nasal alae and the pupils. In a relaxed position, the lips should be slightly parted, with about 1 to 3 mm of the upper teeth visible. The upper lip is slightly anterior to the lower lip, but this orientation lessens with aging.

The "strength" of a face is largely determined by the prominence of the chin relative to the neck. A line from the tip of the nose to the tip of the chin should have a slight inward cant.

Rhytidectomy (Facelift)

■ Anatomy

Vascular Supply

The face has a rich vascular supply. Laterally it is supplied by large fasciocutaneous perforators from three main arterial trunks: the facial, the superficial temporal, and the ophthalmic arteries—all connected by a rich anastomotic network. Medially, the face is supplied by a series of smaller musculocutaneous perforators: the infraorbital, facial, middle jugal, posterior jugal, and submental arteries—again all interconnected by rich anastomotic networks. The venous system mimics the arterial system and is similarly well connected and redundant. Because of its rich vascular supply, it is difficult to devascularize facial soft tissues.

Soft Tissue Layers

There are five layers of critical anatomy in the face: **skin, subcutaneous fat, the superficial musculoaponeurotic system (SMAS)/muscular layer, a thin layer of fascia, and the facial nerve**. These five layers are consistent in all layers of the face, although in some areas, like the zygomatic arch, the layers can become quite compressed. Correct identification of the five layers of the face keeps surgeons out of trouble.

The SMAS layer is the most heterogeneous. It is fibrous, muscular, or fatty, depending on the location in the face. The muscles of facial expression are part of the SMAS layer, and these muscles are innervated by the facial nerve from their deep surfaces. The SMAS is contiguous with the temporoparietal fascia in the forehead and the platysma muscle in the neck (Figure 10-1).

The **facial nerve** runs deep to the SMAS, innervating the muscles of facial expression (frontalis, orbicularis oculi, zygomaticus major and minor, and platysma) from their deep surfaces. Thus, dissection superficial to the SMAS is safe in terms of protecting the facial nerve; dissection deep to the SMAS requires care. As the branches of the facial nerve run medially, they become more superficial. This is why surgeons who dissect in the sub-SMAS plane laterally change surgical planes at the border of the zygomaticus major to become more superficial.

Retaining Ligaments

The zygomatic ligament and the mandibular ligament anchor the skin of the cheek to underlying bone. They are important because they restrain the skin against gravitational changes at these two points, delineating structures such as the anterior border of the jowl and the nasolabial crease. They are released during rhytidectomy in order to adequately redrape the skin.

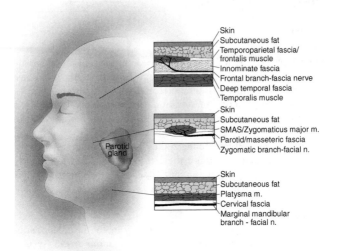

Skin
Subcutaneous fat
Temporoparietal fascia/frontalis muscle
Innominate fascia
Frontal branch-fascia nerve
Deep temporal fascia
Temporalis muscle

Skin
Subcutaneous fat
SMAS/Zygomaticus major m.
Parotid/masseteric fascia
Zygomatic branch-facial n.

Parotid gland

Skin
Subcutaneous fat
Platysma m.
Cervical fascia
Marginal mandibular branch - facial n.

Figure 10-1 • Soft tissue planes of the face.

■ Surgical Technique

Subcutaneous Rhytidectomy

Subcutaneous facelift, the grandfather of techniques, is ideal for young patients with a strong facial skeleton, a thin neck, and a well-defined chin. It does not address the force of gravity on the deeper soft tissues of the face. However, because the plane of dissection is superficial to the facial nerve, it is a safer operation.

A standard facelift incision (Figure 10-2) gives access to the subcutaneous plane. Subcutaneous dissection is carried medially to the lateral orbital rim, 1 cm lateral to the oral commissure, and to the level of the thyroid cartilage. The zygomatic and mandibular ligaments are released so that the tension of the closure is transmitted to the soft tissue of the cheek and jaw, respectively. The skin flap is elevated in a cephaloposterior direction and fixed at two key points: the temporal scalp and the apex of the postauricular incision. Excess skin and subcutaneous tissue are excised and the wound is closed.

SMAS Rhytidectomy

Most patients seeking a facelift have extensive submental fat pads, platysmal banding, and jowls, which are best treated by mobilizing the SMAS in addition to skin flaps. The SMAS can be elevated and plicated as a separate layer or along with skin flaps.

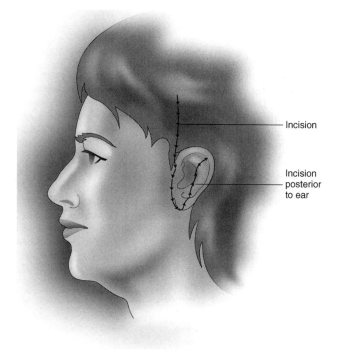

Figure 10-2 • Standard facelift incision.

The rationale for SMAS rhytidectomy is that the stronger, sturdier SMAS transmits a longer-lasting suspensory pull on the facial tissues. The SMAS layer is pulled in a cephaloposterior direction similar to skin flaps in the classic facelift. A thorough understanding of facial nerve anatomy is an important safety concern for this procedure.

Subperiosteal Rhytidectomy

Subperiosteal facelift is a relatively new technique in which the surgeon elevates a flap containing all soft tissues of the face off of the lateral facial skeleton. The soft tissue flap is pulled in a cephaloposterior direction, and the periosteum is tacked in its new position. The muscles of facial expression actually change vectors because their lateral origins are moved. Proponents of the subperiosteal facelift claim that moving the mimetic muscles elevates the corner of the mouth and relieves oral "frowning." Critics claim that the technique provides inadequate redraping of the skin, leaving patients with significant wrinkling in the cheek, perioral region, and neck. Although the plane of dissection is deep to the plane of the facial nerve, the surgeon must be aware of its position at all times.

■ Complications

Hematomas are the most frequent complication of facelift surgery, occurring about 2% of the time. The risk for hematomas is twice as high in men. Their etiology is multifactorial and is associated with inadequate hemostasis, postoperative hypertension, and vomiting. Treatment ranges from surgical drainage, to percutaneous needle aspiration, to watchful waiting depending on the size and location of the hematoma.

The most commonly injured nerve during a facelift is the great auricular nerve, causing lack of sensation over a portion of the ear and scalp. Permanent facial nerve palsy occurs in less than 1% of patients undergoing rhytidectomy. The buccal branch of the facial nerve is the most frequently injured branch, followed by the marginal mandibular and the temporal branches. When recognized intraoperatively, nerves are meticulously repaired. Sub-SMAS facelifts have a slightly higher rate of facial nerve injury than subcutaneous facelifts.

Skin slough is most common in the postauricular area, and usually leads to more noticeable scars. Incidence is about 1% to 3%, with higher rates associated with smoking, hematoma, infection, and excessive tension on the skin closure. It is usually treated conservatively.

Other minor complications of facelifts include hair loss, hypertrophic scarring, skin paresthesias, earlobe deformities, and infection. Fortunately, they occur rarely, and most are treated conservatively.

Browlift

■ Anatomy

The temporal branch of the facial nerve innervates the muscles of the forehead, specifically the frontalis, corrugators, procerus, and superior portion of the orbicularis oculi. The sensory nerves to the forehead are the supraorbital and supratrochlear nerves, both of which exit foramina on the superomedial aspect of the orbit with the supraorbital nerve running lateral to the supratrochlear nerve.

The paired frontalis muscles extend from the galea aponeurotica to the orbicularis oculi muscles and act to elevate the brow and forehead. The depressors of the brow and forehead are the procerus, corrugator supercilii, depressor supercilii, and orbicularis oculi muscles. The paired procerus muscles are oriented vertically along the medial brow and produce transverse wrinkling at the nasal root. The paired corrugators are oriented obliquely from superolaterally to inferomedially to produce vertical wrinkling at the nasal root.

A lifetime of activity of forehead and upper facial musculature results in transverse forehead wrinkles, glabellar wrinkles, transverse and vertical folds at the root of the nose, a lowering of the position of the brow, and upper eyelid fullness.

■ Surgical Technique

Coronal (Direct) Technique

The goals of surgery are to elevate the brow to a more youthful position and remove wrinkles of the transverse forehead, glabellum, and root of the nose. The direct technique uses a coronal incision extending from ear to ear approximately 7 to 9 cm behind the anterior hairline. From this incision, a flap of skin and subcutaneous tissue is elevated in the areolar plane between the galea and the pericranium to the level of the brow, taking care to identify and preserve the supraorbital and supratrochlear nerves. Part or all of the corrugators and procerus muscles are transected, and the flap is redraped to position the brow. Excess skin and subcutaneous tissue are excised with transposition of the anterior hairline posteriorly, a negative in patients with an already high hairline. Care is taken to avoid excessive lift, which may create a "frightened" appearance. The coronal technique is useful in older patients with extensive forehead and glabellar wrinkles, as well as a low-set anterior hairline.

Endoscopic Technique

The endoscopic approach allows access to the forehead and brow through small coronal incisions for release of the retaining structures of the upper face. Forehead and brow dissection are carried out under endoscopic visualization in a manner similar to the coronal technique. The procerus and corrugators are transected, and some form of fixation from brow to scalp provides a lift. The endoscopic technique is useful in younger patients with fewer transverse forehead wrinkles and moderate brow ptosis.

■ Complications

Forehead and brow lifts have low complication rates. Hematomas are rare, but the procedure could conceivably cause orbital hematomas or soft tissue ischemia. Alopecia and infection are similarly uncommon. Paralysis of the frontalis muscle is rare due to plane of dissection. Forehead numbness caused by division of either the supratrochlear or supraorbital nerves is avoided with careful dissection.

Blepharoplasty

The eye is a focal point of human interaction. Thus, facial rejuvenation often begins with the eyes.

■ Anatomy

Eyelid skin is the thinnest in the body and abruptly transitions to the thick malar skin. The palpebral fissure measures around 3 cm in length and extends from medial to lateral canthal tendon. On neutral forward gaze, the lower eyelid rests at the edge of the iris while the upper eyelid covers the upper 2 mm of the upper edge of the iris. Tarsal plates border the upper and lower eyelids, providing support for the soft tissues. White individuals have a well-developed supratarsal fold which Asians lack.

The orbicularis oculi muscle is the eyelid sphincter. A broad, oval muscle, it attaches to the medial canthal tendon, the frontal bone, the lateral canthus, and the inferomedial orbital margin. It is innervated by branches of the facial nerve, and acts to close the eyelids. The levator palpebrae superioris muscle raises the upper eyelid, originating from the lesser wing of the sphenoid and inserting on the tarsus.

The orbital septum is a dense fibroelastic band that forms the anterior border of the orbital contents. Posterior to it in both the upper and lower eyelid are fat pads that can herniate over time, giving the eyelids a full appearance. Anterior to the orbital septum lie fat pads that can also droop with time to cause baggy eyelids. The lacrimal gland lies in the lateral portion of the upper lid. It is uncommonly mistaken for intraorbital fat and resected, leading to inadequate tear production.

■ Pathophysiology

- **Blepharochalasis** is a rare inherited disorder of childhood characterized by repetitive episodes of eyelid edema that eventually lead to attenuation or dehiscence of the levator aponeurosis with resultant drooping of the eyelid (ptosis).
- **Dermatochalasis** is the stretching and involution of the skin and soft tissue of the eyelids that occurs over a lifetime.
- **Steatoblepharon** is puffiness of fat that is either excessive or protruding through a lax septum.
- **Blepharoptosis** is drooping of the upper eyelid. Drooping of the upper eyelid caused by abnormal lowering of the brow is termed **pseudoblepharoptosis**.

■ Preoperative Evaluation

Preoperative evaluation for blepharoplasty focuses on ocular history, ocular and periocular anatomy, ocular function, Schirmer's testing, and tear film breakup time. The history includes use of glasses or contact lenses, symptoms of dry eyes, neuropathy, presence of endocrine disorders including diabetes, glaucoma, and any prior facial surgery. Standard examination of extraocular eye movements, pupillary function, and fundoscopic examination are complemented by the "snap back test," which tests skin turgor. Schirmer's testing and tear film breakup time are measures of a patient's tear quality and tear clearance apparatus. Levator excursion, the primary determinant of eyelid ptosis, is measured from downgaze to upgaze while blocking the brow.

■ Surgical Technique

Classically, blepharoplasty has involved resection of excess skin, fat, and orbicularis muscle from the upper and lower eyelids. Through upper lid incisions, excess skin, fat, and muscle have been excised from several millimeters above the tarsus to just below the brow. Lower lid resection of skin and muscle occurs in an elliptical fashion at the lid margin. Small openings in the orbital septum have facilitated removal of excess herniated fat.

Current techniques in blepharoplasty have focused on redraping orbital contents rather than their resection. Such techniques evolved in response to earlier results, which left patients with a "skeletal" appearance from resection of orbital fat and soft tissue.

■ Complications

Blindness caused by **acute orbital hemorrhage** occurs in less than 1% of patients. Corneal injury can occur, but is minimized by the use of corneal shields. Eyelid **ptosis** can occur postoperatively if the levator aponeurosis is injured. Thus, any injury of the levator must be repaired immediately. **Lagophthalmos**, or eyelid retraction leading to corneal exposure, occurs to some degree in many patients in the early postoperative period. It is well tolerated in the short-term with normal tear production. Persistent lagophthalmos may require surgical correction with a full-thickness skin graft. **Ectropion**, or an abnormal outward cant to the lower lid, is a common, devastating complication of blepharoplasty. Mild cases of ectropion may be treated conservatively in the acute period. However, progressive degrees of lid retraction must be addressed surgically.

Rhinoplasty

■ Anatomy

The nasal pyramid consists of thick, glaborous skin overlying an osseocartilaginous framework. It can be divided roughly into

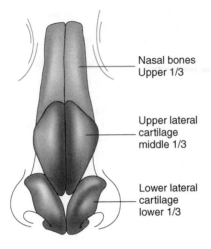

Figure 10-3 • The nose.

thirds with the upper third containing the paired nasal bones, the middle third containing the upper lateral cartilages, and the lower third containing the tip–lobule complex (Figure 10-3). Alternatively, the nose can be divided into its four "aesthetic units": the nasion, the dorsum, the tip, and the base.

The nasal septum arises from the perpendicular plate of the ethmoid bone, vomer, and maxilla, and provides support to the nasal dorsum, upper lateral cartilages and lower lateral cartilages. The turbinates and nasal "valves" (internal and external) act as "resistors" to air flow.

The nose has a rich vascular supply originating from the facial artery, the dorsal nasal branch of the ophthalmic artery, and the infraorbital branch of the maxillary artery. The tip is supplied mainly by the angular artery, a branch of the lateral nasal artery. Veins drain into the ophthalmic and anterior facial veins. Sensation is derived from the maxillary division of the trigeminal nerve.

■ **Initial Evaluation**

The rhinoplasty consultation elucidates a patient's aesthetic and functional complaints. The most frequent aesthetic complaints are a large dorsal hump, an unattractive tip, and a nose that is too wide. Patients often complain of difficulty breathing through one or both nostrils, a manifestation of a deviated septum, hypertrophied turbinates, collapse of the nasal "valves" with inspiration, or a combination of these.

The four external aesthetic areas of the nose—the radix, dorsum, tip, and base—are inspected in front of a large mirror, with patient and surgeon focusing on potential areas of change. Next, the surgeon examines the internal nose with a nasal speculum and headlight. Attention is directed to external and internal nasal valves during inspiration and expiration, the nasal septum, the turbinates, and the nasal mucosa. The Cottle maneuver, wherein the surgeon relieves collapse of the internal nasal valve by lateral retraction on the cheek, determines whether cartilaginous "spreader" grafts between the nasal septum and the upper lateral cartilages will improve airflow in the nasal airway.

During the consultation, the surgeon and patient develop rapport and a surgical plan. Preoperative photographs are taken as well. It is important for the patient to be comfortable with the surgeon; similarly, it is the surgeon's duty to feel comfortable with the patient's motives for pursing rhinoplasty. A patient with an unrealistic understanding of self and unrealistic operative expectations may suffer from psychological disease to which surgery is not the answer.

■ Surgical Technique

There are unlimited techniques to produce a satisfying rhinoplasty. Selection of technique is based on surgeon preference and experience, and the patient's goals.

Surgical Approach

There are two basic operative approaches to the external nose: the open approach and the closed approach. The **open approach** consists of transcolumellar and bilateral marginal incisions, which allow the soft tissue overlying the nasal tip to be elevated, exposing the cartilaginous framework. This approach is popular due to a shorter learning curve and wide access to all structures of the nose.

The **closed approach** consists of a combination of incisions in the nasal mucosa, either around, or in between the cartilages. **Intercartilaginous incisions** are located in between upper lateral and lower lateral cartilages. Intracartilaginous incisions go through the lower lateral cartilages. Infracartilaginous incisions follow the caudal border of the lower lateral cartilages. The closed approach offers limited visibility and flexibility, requiring wisdom on the part of the surgeon. On the other hand, its simplicity, speed of dissection, and absence of external incisions have made it popular among surgeons and patients alike.

The Nasal Dorsum

The nasal dorsum is a focal point of patient dissatisfaction. Reduction of the nasal dorsum is a classic maneuver, while dorsal augmentation has recently gained favor. The position and volume of the nasal dorsum can be changed via osteotomy followed by outfracture or infracture of nasal bones, resection of bone and cartilage, or rasping of bone and cartilage. Width and height can be added to the nasal dorsum using cartilage onlay grafts, cartilage spreader grafts, alloplastic implants, and alloderm. The nasofrontal angle is inevitably changed by the above maneuvers.

The Tip–Lobule Complex

The shape and position of the lower lateral (alar) cartilages determines the outline of the tip–lobule complex. Thus, changes to the alar cartilages cause the most dramatic changes in the character of the tip–lobule complex. Repositioning, crushing or scoring, partial resection, suturing the paired alar cartilages together in various conformations, and a multitude of grafting techniques have all been applied to tip surgery. Long-term results of surgery of the tip–lobule complex are among the most unpredictable.

■ Complications

Acute complications following rhinoplasty include hemorrhage or hematoma, septal perforation, infection, anesthetic-related problems, and failure of the repair. Late complications include excessive scarring, vestibular webbing, persistence of edema, and failure to meet the aesthetic goals of the patient.

Otoplasty

■ Diagnosis

The most common causes of a prominent ear are overdeveloped conchal bowl and underdeveloped antihelical fold. Both conditions produce an ear that protrudes excessively from the temporal skull, attracting unwanted attention.

■ Treatment

The shape of the auricular cartilage can be altered by altering the position of the cartilage, altering the intrinsic shape of the cartilage, or excising cartilage. Placement of Mustarde sutures from the conchal bowl to the mastoid periosteum decreases the depth of the conchal bowl. Similarly, placing sutures from the upper auricular pole to the temporal scalp decreases the prominence of the helix and creates a more prominent antihelical fold. Cutting or abrading cartilage releases intrinsic stresses, causing it to bend away from the side that is cut or abraded. Abrading the auricular cartilage's anterior surface will produce a more acute auriculo-cephalic angle, thus making the ears less prominent.

Body Contouring and Liposuction

Body contouring and liposuction are among the most commonly performed aesthetic operations in the world. They improve the appearance of various areas of the body through fat aspiration or resection, musculofascial plication, and skin resection. Common reasons for consultation include recent weight fluctuation (gain or loss), postpartum changes in body contour, and dissatisfaction with body habitus.

Interestingly, there has been an explosive increase in patients seeking body contouring after losing massive amounts of weight (usually via bariatric surgery). These patients commonly present with abdominal wall hernias and massive amounts of excess subcutaneous skin and fat, a challenge for the body contouring surgeon.

■ Liposuction

Liposuction refers to aspiration of subcutaneous fat through small-diameter cannulas under vacuum or ultrasound assistance. Fat adheres to the opening in the distal end of the cannula due to suction from the vacuum, and is then avulsed with a to-and-fro motion. Ultrasound-assisted liposuction (UAL) uses ultrasonic energy to melt subcutaneous fat prior to aspirating it through cannulas. Neurovascular tissue is relatively resistant to vacuum suction and ultrasonic energy, making it relatively resistant to liposuction.

Preoperatively patients are marked topographically to direct fat aspiration. A solution of lidocaine and epinephrine, the so-called "tumescent" or "wetting" solution, is used to thoroughly infiltrate the surgical site. Effective anesthesia and vasospasm is present in 10 minutes, after which the surgeon can safely puncture the skin and insert the cannula into the subcutaneous compartment. The end point of aspiration is determined by the appearance of the treated area and the volume of the aspirate. Postoperatively, patients wear compression garments over the surgical sites to ensure that the overlying skin heals in the correct position.

Serious complications following liposuction are rare. Bleeding, infection, seroma, and hematoma are the most frequent complications, all occurring less than 1% of the time. Postoperative contour irregularities caused by overaspiration or underaspiration are more common, and lead to secondary procedures in 5% to 15% of patients. Skin hyperpigmentation and hypertrophic scarring are rare. Large volume liposuction (greater that 4 liters of aspirate) has been associated with severe fluid shifts. Patients undergoing large volume liposuction should be monitored in the early post-operative period.

■ Abdominoplasty

Abdominoplasty treats excess skin, excess subcutaneous fat, and abdominal wall laxity. The classic abdominoplasty is an elliptical excision of infraumbilical soft tissue, umbilical transposition, and abdominal wall fascial plication. In essence, abdominoplasty is an advancement flap closure of a lower abdominal soft tissue defect based on the superficial and deep epigastric arteries and the lateral intercostal artery perforators. Most surgeons flex the operating table, which in turn flexes the patient's torso, to gain a mechanical advantage on a tight closure. Closure under tension renders the "tip" of the advancement flap ischemic, and about 3% of the time the wound edges undergo frank necrosis. Most surgeons leave drains beneath the skin flaps to lessen the risk for developing a seroma or hematoma.

■ Torsoplasty

Torsoplasty refers to combining abdominoplasty with a similar excision of lower back subcutaneous tissue and skin, forming a ring of excised tissue circumferentially that is closed using advancement flaps. Torsoplasty is indicated in individuals with the combination of a large abdominal pannus and large flank fat rolls.

■ Brachioplasty and Thigh Lifts

Patients seeking body contouring often complain of excess soft tissue in the upper arms and thighs. Patients without large amounts of excess skin may see dramatic improvement with liposuction alone. The majority have excess skin and subcutaneous tissue, necessitating elliptical excision along the medial arm and medial thigh. Because of the location, hypertrophic scarring is not uncommon. Hematomas and seromas are common as well.

A Opportunities in Plastic Surgery

Jesse A. Taylor, MD

Plastic and reconstructive surgery is a field of enormous breadth. After training, a plastic surgeon is equipped with many tools; deciding how to apply those tools further defines the plastic surgeon. There are plastic surgeons who prefer the art of aesthetic surgery, and who perform all of their operations in an outpatient surgery center on a fee-for-service basis. Others choose to practice pediatric craniofacial surgery, a field that requires a team of specialists rarely found outside tertiary care centers. Still others migrate toward the field of hand surgery, rarely venturing beyond the hand and forearm. What is the common thread that binds? All are surgeons who strive to restore form and function so that their patients can live happy lives.

There are a variety of ways to become a board-certified plastic surgeon. The traditional approach involves completing a residency in general surgery, or one of the surgical specialties, followed by a fellowship in plastic surgery (2 clinical years). Over the past 30 years, the "combined" or "integrated" training approach has gained in popularity. These trainees spend 6 years training in both general and plastic surgery, 3 years of each. Additionally, dentists with oromaxillofacial surgery training may become plastic surgeons through a variety of channels. The common denominator in all these approaches is a dedicated period of 2 to 3 years of training in an ACGME accredited plastic surgery training program. Training is followed by both oral and written board examinations, the passage of which confers board certification. Additional information about plastic surgery training opportunities can be found on the Internet at **www.sfmatch.org** and the National Residency Matching Program's (NRMP's) website (**www.nrmp.org**).

The five major subspecialties within the field of plastic and reconstructive surgery are aesthetic surgery, hand and microvascular surgery, breast surgery, burn surgery, and craniofacial surgery. Fellowships in each of these areas are available following completion of a general plastic surgery training program.

B Review Questions and Answers

QUESTIONS

1. A 24-year-old woman presents with tenderness, swelling, and edema of the palmar tip of her dominant index finger. She suffered a puncture wound to that area about 6 days prior to presentation. What is the most appropriate next step in management?

   A. Observation
   B. Antibiotics
   C. Splinting
   D. Incision and drainage
   E. Excision and grafting

2. What is the theoretical gain in length with a Z-plasty using 60 degree angles?

   A. 25%
   B. 40%
   C. 75%
   D. 90%
   E. 120%

3. A 53-year-old farmer seeks consultation for a wound on his nose that has been present for over 2 years and seems to be growing. He has noted intermittent bleeding in the past. On physical examination, the lesion is a nonpigmented ulcer with pearly borders, it measures less than 1 cm in diameter, and it is covered with a scab-like material. There is no palpable cervical lymphadenopathy. What is the next step in management?

   A. MRI
   B. Biopsy
   C. Wide local excision
   D. Electrodesiccation
   E. Topical 5-fluorouracil

4. The most common skin cancer is which of the following?

   A. Squamous cell carcinoma
   B. Merkel cell carcinoma
   C. Basal cell carcinoma
   D. Melanoma
   E. Kaposi's sarcoma

5. A 23-year-old African-American woman presents complaining of an abnormally large scar on her right earlobe that has developed over the past year. She began to notice this growth about 1 month after having her ear pierced, and has noted continued growth in the ensuing months. The lesion now measures $3 \times 4 \times 5$ cm, centered about the lobule of her right ear. Which of the following therapies is a recognized method of treating her problem?

   A. Immunosuppression
   B. Cryodesiccation
   C. Thermal injury
   D. Intralesional corticosteroid injection
   E. Intralesional antibiotic injection

6. The optimal treatment of asymptomatic hemangiomas early in childhood is which of the following?

   A. Immunosuppression
   B. Electrocautery
   C. Cryodesiccation
   D. Observation
   E. Excision

7. A 33-year-old man is involved in a motorcycle accident that has resulted in a liver laceration, a mild concussion, and a Gustilo IIIb tibial plateau fracture (proximal tibial fracture). His foot is sensate, and he has approximately 8 cm of exposed tibia just below his knee. His lower extremity musculature appears injured anteriorly; his posterior compartments appear intact. What is the most commonly used reconstructive option for bony coverage in this patient?

   A. Soleus muscle flap
   B. Skin graft
   C. Gastrocnemius muscle flap
   D. Free tissue transfer
   E. Healing by secondary intention

8. The latissimus dorsi muscle flap is based on the:

   A. Long thoracic artery
   B. Superior epigastric artery
   C. Internal mammary artery
   D. Thoracodorsal artery
   E. Lateral thoracic artery

9. Which of the following cell types is most critical during the inflammatory phase of wound healing?

   A. Mast cells
   B. Macrophages
   C. Langerhans' cells
   D. PMNs
   E. Lymphocytes

10. A 75-year-old man with advanced chronic obstructive pulmonary disease (COPD) from a lifetime of smoking, on home oxygen therapy, sustains extensive burns to the head and neck while trying to smoke a cigarette with his nasal cannula oxygen in place. He is brought to the emergency department where he is noted to be breathing 40 times a minute with oxygen saturations of 92%. He is producing a copious amount of carbonaceous sputum and has blackish nasal hairs and eyebrows. While you are talking to the patient, he becomes unresponsive and his oxygen saturation drops to 82%. What is the appropriate initial step in management?

    A. Chest compressions
    B. Intubation
    C. Inspection of burn wounds
    D. Escharotomy
    E. Administration of IV fluids

11. The Ehlers-Danlos syndrome is characterized by:

    A. Lax, pebbled skin with subcutaneous calcium deposition
    B. Premature aging
    C. Hypermobile joints and fragile skin due to abnormal collagen cross-linking
    D. Cutaneous papules

12. A 29-year-old African-American woman presents to your office complaining of back pain and breast strap notching due to large, pendulous breasts. She desires reduction mammaplasty. Which of the following is a recognized complication of reduction mammaplasty?

    A. Loss of nipple sensation
    B. Reduced ability to breast-feed
    C. Unsightly scars
    D. Wound infection
    E. All of the above

13. According to the Parkland formula, a 70-kg man with a 30% TBSA burn would receive how much fluid in the first 8 hours of resuscitation?

    A. 3,200 mL
    B. 3,600 mL
    C. 3 800 mL
    D. 4,200 mL

14. What is the leading cause of morbidity and mortality due to burns?

    A. Inhalation injury
    B. Hyperthermia
    C. Infection
    D. Metabolic derangements

15. A 53-year-old woman who works as a transcriptionist presents to your office with symptoms of pain, paresthesia, hypesthesia, or

numbness in the thumb, index finger, long finger, and radial aspect of the ring finger. She also complains of pain and numbness that awakens her from sleep in the middle of the night. Activities that require prolonged wrist flexion or gripping (driving a car, typing) sometimes aggravate her symptoms. She manifests pain in her fingertips when you tap on her volar wrist. What is her diagnosis?

A. Cubital tunnel syndrome
B. Carpal tunnel syndrome
C. Dupuytren's disease
D. Flexor tenosynovitis
E. Posterior interosseus nerve syndrome

16. Which of the following lower extremity soft tissue injuries is correctly matched with its typical reconstructive option?

A. Foot—gastrocnemius flap
B. Middle third of tibia—soleus muscle flap
C. Proximal third of tibia—free flap
D. Thigh—soleus muscle flap
E. Distal third of tibia—gastrocnemius muscle flap

17. A 16-year-old girl gives birth to a healthy male baby. Several months after his birth, she begins to notice that his skull has an abnormally increased anteroposterior dimension and decreased width. Her son has which of the following conditions:

A. Trigonocephaly
B. Metopic craniosynostosis
C. Scaphocephaly
D. Brachycephaly
E. Posterior plagiocephaly

18. A 42-year-old woman desires autologous breast reconstruction after mastectomy for stage II breast cancer. Her best option would be:

A. Expander/implant
B. TRAM flap reconstruction
C. No breast reconstruction
D. Latissimus flap over an expander/implant

19. A 55-year-old man seeks consultation for rhytidectomy. He has jowling and prominent platysmal banding, and you believe he would be an excellent candidate for a facelift. Which of the following complications occurs more commonly in men than in women?

A. Skin loss
B. Infection
C. Facial nerve injury
D. Injury to the greater auricular nerve
E. Hematoma

20. A 44-year-old man has a burn scar contracture in his right antecubital fossa that limits his ability to straighten his elbow. Which of the

following types of skin grafts would be most appropriate for use in a contracture release?

A. Full-thickness skin graft
B. Thick split-thickness skin graft
C. Medium-thickness split-thickness skin graft
D. Thin split-thickness skin graft
E. Ultradelicate split-thickness skin graft

21. A 21-year-old IV drug abuser presents to the emergency room with a superficial abscess of the volar forearm. The abscess is surrounded by minimal erythematous skin. The patient has had no fevers. What is the appropriate definitive treatment for this problem?

A. Oral antibiotics
B. Intravenous antibiotics
C. Incision and drainage
D. Insertion of a percutaneous drain at the wound site
E. Observation

22. When a wound is fully healed, its tensile strength is approximately what percentage of its original strength?

A. 50%
B. 60%
C. 70%
D. 80%
E. 90%

23. Which of the following is a cardinal sign of flexor tenosynovitis?

A. Finger held in extension
B. Pain in the forearm
C. Pinpoint pain in the finger DIP joint
D. Pain on passive extension

24. Recognized approaches for placement of breast implants for augmentation mammaplasty include which of the following?

A. Suprasternal
B. Inframammary fold
C. Epigastric
D. Parasternal

25. Which branch of the facial nerve is most commonly injured during facelift surgery?

A. Temporal
B. Zygomatic
C. Buccal
D. Marginal mandibular

ANSWER KEY

1. D	10. B	19. E
2. C	11. C	20. A
3. B	12. E	21. C
4. C	13. D	22. D
5. D	14. C	23. D
6. D	15. B	24. B
7. C	16. B	25. C
8. D	17. C	
9. B	18. B	

ANSWERS

1. **D. This patient has a felon, an abscess of the palmar surface of the fingertip. These infections need to be incised and drained, which usually provides the patient with immediate relief.**

2. **C.** Z-plasty is a technique that is often used to correct scar contracture, especially when it affects function. It allows for a gain in length and a change in direction so that mobility improves. All limbs of the "Z" must be equal in length. The angle between limbs can vary from 30 to 90 degrees based on the desired gain in length. **The standard Z-plasty uses 60 degree angles, which gives a 75% increase in length.** The less acute the angle, the greater the gain in length but the more tension placed on the suture line. For example, 30 degree angles produce a 25% gain in length, whereas 90 degree angles produce a 120% gain in length.

3. **B.** Diagnosis must precede treatment. This patient's nonhealing ulcer in a sun-exposed area may represent a malignancy that may require definitive resection or electrodesiccation. **However, prior to proceeding with therapy, the diagnosis must be made. Usually this is done via tissue biopsy.**

4. **C. Basal cell carcinoma (BCC) is the most common skin cancer, accounting for over 75% of cases. Sun exposure is the major risk factor, though prior radiation and immunosuppression also increase the risk.**

5. **D.** The treatment of keloids is difficult. **Surgical reexcision alone has been associated with higher recurrence rates than reexcision combined with local injection of corticosteroids.** For moderately large keloids, the addition of pressure therapy in the form of custom compression wraps and garments helps. Finally, for large, treatment-resistant keloids, the best results are reported with a combination of surgery, **corticosteroid injection**, and postoperative radiotherapy.

6. **D. Most hemangiomas involute and resolve with time. The optimal management of an asymptomatic hemangioma early in childhood is observation.**

7. **C. Due to a paucity of local soft tissue, the knee and proximal tibia are two areas where muscle flaps are frequently required for bony coverage. The workhorse of soft tissue coverage around the knee and proximal tibia are the medial and lateral heads of the gastrocnemius muscle, which can fill a defect up to 9 cm medially and 5 to 7 cm laterally.** One or both these heads can be raised based on the lateral or medial sural arteries, which enter each muscle proximally from their tibial surface. The lesser saphenous vein and sural nerve travel in the cleft between the gastrocnemius muscles and should be preserved when possible. The function of the gastrocnemius is ankle plantar flexion as well as some knee flexion, but its loss is tolerable when the soleus muscle is preserved. Although muscles such as the tibialis anterior are in close proximity to the knee and proximal tibia, these muscles have a segmental blood supply (Mathes and Nahai type IV), cannot be mobilized extensively to cover the defect, and are often in the zone of injury.

8. **D.** The latissimus dorsi muscle originates from the spinous processes of T7–T12 and L1–L5, the sacrum, the posterior superior iliac crest, and ribs 9 through 12 and inserts anteriorly onto the proximal humerus. It is a Mathes and Nahai type V muscle with one dominant pedicle entering the lateral edge of the muscle and several segmental pedicles based on medial perforators. **For breast reconstruction, the LDM is raised as a pedicled flap based on the dominant thoracodorsal neurovascular bundle.**

9. **B. Macrophages are key players in wound healing. They achieve high concentrations in the wound by 48 hours and remain throughout the inflammatory phase of wound healing, actively participating in débridement.** They promote angiogenesis and release chemokines that attract fibroblasts to the wound, thus regulating the synthesis and deposition of collagen.

10. **B. This patient has suffered an inhalational injury and is in respiratory distress. The first step in managing such a patient is intubation.** Treatment of inhalational injury is supportive, and includes the administration of 100% oxygen (which decreases the washout time of CO from 250 minutes to 40–50 minutes). Frequent nasotracheal suctioning of carbonaceous materials to prevent mucous plugging and aggressive treatment of infectious pulmonary complications are also indicated.

11. **C. Cutis hyperelastica is a rare, usually autosomal-dominant disorder characterized by fragile, hyperelastic and easily bruised skin, joint hypermobility, and aortic aneurysm.** Abnormal molecular cross-linking of collagen leads to poor wound healing. The skin has a low tensile strength and does not hold suture material.

Pseudoxanthoma elasticum is an autosomal-recessive disease characterized by increased collagen degradation and deposits of calcium and fat on the elastic fibers. Progeria is characterized by premature aging.

12. **E. Complications of reduction mammaplasty include loss of nipple sensation or erectile function, reduced ability to breast-feed, unsightly scars, wound infection, and recurrence (thus all of the above).** These risks must be weighed against the benefit of reduction for all patients, especially pubertal females. There is controversy as to whether scarring and fat necrosis after breast reduction can lead to mammographic abnormalities that would obscure or confuse the diagnosis of breast cancer. For this reason, many surgeons recommend reference mammograms before and after surgery and a low threshold for biopsy of suspicious lesions.

13. **D. Parkland formula day 1: lactated Ringer's solution: total volume = 4 mL/kg/% TBSA burn. Give half in first 8 hours; give half over the next 16 hours. Therefore, a 70-kg male with 30% TBSA burns should receive 4 mL × 70 kg × 30% = 8,400 mL of lactated Ringer's solution in the first day of the Parkland formula. Half of the 8,400 mL (i.e., 4,200 mL) should be given over the first 8 hours of treatment.**

14. **C.** With improvement in ICU care and the philosophy of early excision and grafting of wounds, the percentage of patients who die acutely from thermal injury has decreased significantly over the past 30 years. Death during early recovery, largely due to sepsis, remains a challenge. **Infection continues to be the leading cause of morbidity and mortality overall, with pulmonary infection the usual source.**

15. **B. This patient suffers from carpal tunnel syndrome, or compression of the median nerve as it courses through the carpal tunnel of the volar wrist. Her symptoms of pain and paresthesia in the thumb, index, long, and radial ring fingers is classic. She also has a positive Tinel's sign, another classic feature of carpal tunnel syndrome.** Further workup would entail EMG/NCVs.

16. **B.** Defects of the muscular thigh typically require simple advancement of local muscles to cover an exposed femur and a split-thickness skin graft to replace missing skin. The workhorse of soft tissue coverage around the knee and proximal tibia are the medial and lateral heads of the gastrocnemius muscle. **The middle third of the tibia classically is covered by a soleus or hemisoleus muscle flap.** Because there are no suitable muscle flaps that can be rotated to cover wounds in the distal tibia or the foot, free flaps are often needed for exposed bone, joint, or tendon.

17. **C. The baby has scaphocephaly (boat-shaped skull), a condition caused by premature fusion of the sagittal suture. Scaphocephaly is the most common single-suture craniosynostosis.**

18. **B.** This patient would be best served by a TRAM flap (either pedicled or free). The TRAM flap is the most commonly used flap for breast reconstruction, and is the only choice from above to use only autologous tissue.

19. **E.** Hematomas are the most frequent complication of facelift surgery, occurring around 1% to 3% of the time. The risk for hematomas is twice as high in men as it is in women. Their etiology is multifactorial, and is associated with inadequate hemostasis, postoperative hypertension, and vomiting. Treatment ranges from surgical drainage, to percutaneous needle aspiration, to watchful waiting depending on the size and location of the hematoma. Other complications of rhytidectomy including skin loss, infection, facial nerve injury, and greater auricular nerve injury occur without sex predilection.

20. **A.** Full-thickness skin grafts undergo the least amount of secondary contraction. Thus, a full-thickness skin graft would be the best candidate for releasing this patient's burn scar contracture.

21. **C.** Proper treatment of a superficial upper extremity abscess is incision and drainage. Additional therapy may consist of oral or intravenous antibiotics depending on the amount of cellulitis present. However, antibiotics are not the answer to this problem. It would not be wise to insert a percutaneous drain or observe this process either.

22. **D.** Under ideal conditions, the maximal tensile strength of a wound is approximately 80% of its premorbid tensile strength. A wound reaches its maximal tensile strength by 6 weeks into the healing process.

23. **D.** The cardinal signs of flexor tenosynovitis, as described by Kanavel, are fusiform swelling of the finger, pain with passive extension, tenderness over tendon sheath, and flexed position of the finger. It is important to diagnose this aggressive infection early so that surgical débridement can be performed prior to flexor tendon incapacitation.

24. **B.** The choice of incision for implant placement is a balance between exposure of the surgical site and a well-hidden scar. The inframammary fold incision was the first to be described, and it is still the most widely used. Other incisions include the periareolar, the transaxillary, the transareolar, and the transumbilical.

25. **C.** The most commonly injured nerve during a facelift is the great auricular nerve, causing lack of sensation over a portion of the ear and scalp. Permanent facial nerve palsy occurs in less than 1% of patients undergoing rhytidectomy. Sub-SMAS facelifts have a slightly higher rate than subcutaneous facelifts. The buccal branch of the facial nerve is the most frequently injured branch, followed by the marginal mandibular and the temporal branches. When recognized intraoperatively, nerves are meticulously repaired.

C Commonly Prescribed Medications

Ryan Katz, MD

Local Anesthetics

Diffuse into the nerve in uncharged state; become charged and block sodium channels producing local analgesia.

Esters	Onset	Potency	Duration (hr)	Maximum Dose (mg/kg)
Procaine	Rapid	Weak	0.5–1.5	15
Chloroprocaine	Rapid	Weak	0.5–1	15
Tetracaine	Slow	Potent	4–12	2.5
Cocaine	Rapid	Potent	1–2	Topical

Amides	Onset	Potency	Duration (hr)	Maximum Dose (mg/kg)
Lidocaine	Intermediate	Intermediate	1–2	4–5
Mepivacaine	Intermediate	Intermediate	1.5–3	5
Prilocaine	Intermediate	Intermediate	1–2	7
Bupivacaine	Slow	Potent	4–12	2.5
Ropivacaine	Slow	Potent	4–12	2
Etidocaine	Slow	Potent	4–12	5
EMLA cream (prilocaine/lidocaine)	Slow	Intermediate	1–2	

Notes:
- **Esters** are hydrolyzed in the plasma by pseudocholinesterase. A by-product of this reaction is para-amino-benzoic-acid (PABA). Some people are allergic to PABA and should therefore avoid ester-based local anesthetics. These same people should also buy PABA-free sun block.
- **Amides** are metabolized in the liver; true allergy to amides is rare.
- **Cocaine** is the only known local anesthetic that causes vasoconstriction; commonly used as a 4% topical solution in nasal surgery.

- **CNS toxicity**: As the dose approaches toxic levels (or if accidentally injected intravascularly), patients may experience tinnitus, metallic taste, blurred vision, perioral numbness and tingling, or confusion. Ultimately they may have twitching, tonic-clonic seizures, loss of consciousness, or respiratory depression.
- **Cardiovascular toxicity**: At toxic levels, these drugs may cause prolongation of the PR and QRS intervals or malignant arrhythmias (bupivacaine is often noted for its ability to cause recalcitrant arrhythmias).

Antibiotics

	Pathogen	Treatment	Notes
Abscess	***Staphylococcus aureus*** ***Streptococcus*** Gram negative rods Anaerobes	**Broad-spectrum penicillin** Amoxicillin/ clavulanate (augmentin) Piperacillin/ tazobactam (Zosyn)	Incision, drainage, and thorough débridement is the treatment; antibiotics are adjunctive and help treat accompanying cellulitis. Oral therapy is only recommended in uncomplicated infection without fever or sepsis. Strongly consider hospital admission for the diabetic or immunocompromised patient. IV drug abusers have high incidence of MRSA; if MRSA suspected, start vancomycin in addition to your gram-negative or anaerobic coverage.
Burns/eschars	*Staphylococcus* species *Streptococcus* species *Pseudomonas* species	Topical antimicrobials (see Chapter 5)	See Chapter 5
Cat bite/ dog bite	*Staphylococcus* species *Streptococcus* species *Pasteurella multocida*	Amoxicillin/ clavulanate (augmentin)	Must thoroughly washout and débride. Rule out joint involvement.

	Pathogen	Treatment	Notes
Cellulitis	Group A *Streptococcus* *S. aureus*	Nafcillin or oxacillin First-generation cephalosporins	In a diabetic or immunocompromised patient, consider broadening the spectrum of coverage to include gram negatives and anaerobes (piperacillin/tazobactam [Zosyn]). If MRSA suspected, start vancomycin.
Fracture (open)	*S. aureus* *Streptococcus* Gram negatives	First-generation cephalosporin + aminoglycoside (gentamycin) or quinolone (ciprofloxacin)	Must thoroughly wash out and débride. Often polymicrobial contamination. Give tetanus prophylaxis if not up to date or unsure of vaccine status. Antibiotic coverage may be broadened to include gram negatives.
Herpetic whitlow	Herpes simplex virus	Acyclovir	Must thoroughly wash out and débride.
Human bite	*Streptococcus viridans* *S. aureus* *Eikinella corrodens* Anaerobes	Amoxacillin/clavulanate (augmentin)	If the wound appears infected, use broad-spectrum antibiotics like piperacillin/tazobactam (Zosyn) or ampicillin/sulbactam (Unasyn) *Salmonella* osteomyelitis is associated with sickle cell disease.
Osteomyelitis	*S. aureus*	Nafcillin or oxacillin	May require removal of nail to adequately drain.
Paronychia (acute)	*S. aureus* Anaerobes	Clindamycin	Seen in people whose hands are chronically immersed in water (dish washers).
Paronychia (chronic)	*Candida*	Clotrimazole (topical)	Oral therapy with itraconazole may be of some benefit.

	Pathogen	Treatment	Notes
Felon/hand abscess	*S. aureus*	First-generation cephalosporin or dicloxacillin	In a diabetic or immuno-compromised patient, think about broadening the spectrum of coverage to include gram negatives and anaerobes (piperacillin/tazobactam [Zosyn]).
Superficial skin infection or perioperative prophylaxis	Gram positives/skin flora (*Staphylococcus/Streptococcus*)	First-generation cephalosporin	Clindamycin is a good alternative if the patient has a known penicillin or cephalosporin allergy.

Analgesics

Opioids	Trade Name	Dose Range	Metabolism	Notes
Codeine		15–60 mg IV/PO/IM/SC every 4–6 hr	Liver Kidney	May be given in elixir form if unable to open mouth.
Fentanyl	Actiq, Duragesic, Sublimaze	25–100 µg IV/IM every 1–2 hr	Liver	Often used in patient-controlled analgesia (PCA); may also be given by transdermal patch (change every 3 days) or lozenge.
Hydromorphone	Dilaudid	2–4 mg PO every 4–6 hr 0.5–2 mg IV/IM/SC every 4–6 hr	Liver Kidney	Often used in PCA.
Meperidine	Demerol	50–150 IV/IM/SC every 3–4 hr	Liver Kidney	Metabolite (Normeperidine) may cause seizures; causes physical dependence; rarely first-line therapy.

Opioids	Trade Name	Dose Range	Metabolism	Notes
Methadone	Dolophine, metha-done	2.5–10 mg PO/IM/SC every 3–8 hr Opioid-dependent patients may take 20–120 mg PO qd	Liver	Used for chronic pain or as an alternative to IV narcotic abuse.
Morphine		2–4 mg IV/SC every 3–4 hr 10 mg PO every 3–4 hr	Liver Kidney	Often used in PCA; also avail-able as rectal suppository; pruritus may be due to hista-mine release.
Oxycodone	Roxicodone, OxyContin, OxyIR	Immediate-release (OxyIR) 2.5–5 mg PO every 6 hr Controlled-release (OxyContin) 10–40 mg PO every 12 hr	Liver	Oxycodone may be given in elixir form; sustained-release form is not available as elixir; sustained-release cap-sules are not to be crushed.
Propoxy-phene	Darvon, Darvon-N	65–100 mg PO every 4 hr	Liver	Used for mild/moderate pain; not to be used in depressed or suicidal patients.

NSAIDs	Trade Name	Dose Range	Metabolism	Notes
Aspirin	Bayer, Ecotrin	325–650 mg PO/PR every 4–6 hr (maximum 4 g/day)	Kidney	Analgesic, antipyretic, and antiplatelet; unless otherwise indicated would not use as first line for pain control; some patients allergic; side effects include tinnitus/hearing loss; renal papillary necrosis; Reye's syndrome

NSAIDs	Trade Name	Dose Range	Metabolism	Notes
Ibuprofen	Advil, Motrin, Nuprin	200–800 mg PO every 6–8 hr	Liver	Available in tablets and suspension
Naproxen	Aleve, Naprosyn, Anaprox	Immediate-release 250–500 mg PO b.i.d. Delayed-release 375–500 mg PO b.i.d. Controlled-release 750–1,000 mg PO qd	Liver	Available as caplet, gel caplet, and suspension
Oxaprozin	Daypro	600–1,200 mg PO qd	Liver	
Ketorolac	Toradol	15–30 mg IV/IM every 6–8 hr 10 mg PO every 4–6 hr Not to exceed 5 days of continuous use Maximum daily dose is 120 mg	Liver	Is the only IV NSAID; may exacerbate renal failure and promote bleeding through platelet inhibition
Celecoxib	Celebrex	200 mg PO qd or 100 mg PO b.i.d.	Liver	Cyclooxygenase-2 (COX-2) inhibitor; offers comparative analgesia to other NSAIDs with some studies showing fewer GI side effects
Rofecoxib	Vioxx	12.5–25 mg PO qd	Plasma	COX-2 inhibitor; offers comparative analgesia to other NSAIDs with some studies showing fewer GI side effects

NSAIDs	Trade Name	Dose Range	Metabolism	Notes
Valdecoxib	Bextra	10 mg PO qd	Plasma	COX-2 inhibitor; offers comparative analgesia to other NSAIDs with some studies showing fewer GI side effects

Opioid/ NSAID	Trade Name	Dose Range	Metabolism	Notes
Acetaminophen	Tylenol	325–650 mg PO every 4–6 hr; maximum daily dose is 4 g	Liver Kidney	
Codeine/ acetaminophen	Tylenol 3	(30/300 mg) 1–2 tablets PO every 4–6 hr	Liver Kidney	Also available as Tylenol 4 60/300 mg tablets
Propoxyphene/ acetaminophen	Darvocet	(50/325 mg) 1–2 tablets PO every 4–6 hr	Liver	Also available in a 100/650 mg tablets
Hydrocodone/ acetaminophen	Lortab	(2.5/500 mg) 1–2 tablets PO every 4–6 hr	Liver Kidney	Also available in 5/500 mg, 7.5/500 mg, and 10/500 mg tablets
Oxycodone/ acetaminophen	Tylox	(5/500 mg) 1 tablet PO every 4–6 hr	Liver	Different formulations of oxycodone/acetaminophen exist, including Percocet and Roxicet

Antagonists (for suspected overdose)	Trade Name	Dose Range	Metabolism	Notes
Naloxone	Narcan	0.4–2.0 mg IV/IM/SC/ ET every 2–3 min	Liver Kidney	Opioid antagonist; use 0.1–0.2 mg increments if opioid dependent to avoid cardiovascular collapse
Flumazenil	Romazicon	0.2 mg IV over 30 sec then 0.3–0.5 mg IV every 30 sec (maximum dose 3 mg in an hour)	Liver Kidney	Used in benzodiazepine overdose; reversal often wears off before benzodiazepines are metabolized; therefore, repeated doses may be needed

Index

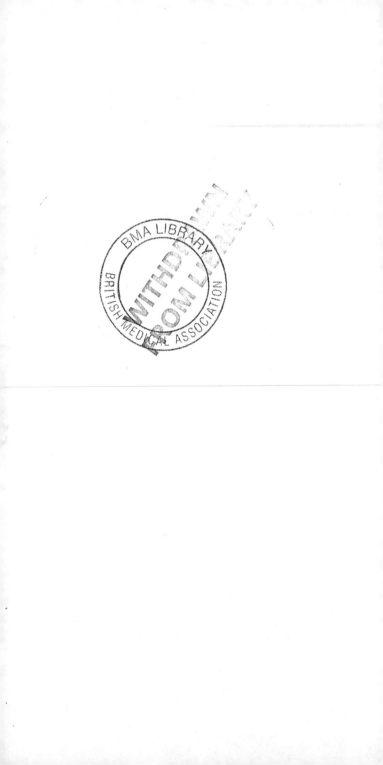